Bipolar disorder
YOUR QUESTIONS ANSWERED

D1236161

For Elsevier

Commissioning Editor: Fiona Conn
Project Development Manager: Isobel Black
Project Manager: Frances Affleck
Designer Direction: George Ajayi
Illustration Manager: Bruce Hogarth
Illustrator: David Graham

How to use this book

The *Your Questions Answered* series aims to meet the information needs of GPs and other primary care professionals who care for patients with chronic conditions. It is designed to help them work with patients and their families, providing effective, evidence-based care and management.

The books are in an accessible question and answer format, with detailed contents lists at the beginning of every chapter and a complete index to help find specific information.

ICONS
Icons are used in the book to identify particular types of information:

 highlights information important to clinical practice

 highlights side-effect information

 highlights case studies which illustrate or help to explain the answers given

PATIENT QUESTIONS
At the end of relevant chapters there are sections of frequently asked patient questions, with easy-to-understand answers aimed at the non-medical reader. These questions are also listed at the end of the book.

What is manic depression (bipolar disorder)?

1

1.1 What is manic depression?

Manic depression is an illness, which has mood changes as the fundamental aspect. Mood disorders are also called affective disorders by those who prefer more technical terms, 'affect' meaning emotion or feeling.

Every illness is characterised by symptoms that are unique in their pattern and also a degree of disability. In psychiatry there is usually also a time course requirement, so that having symptoms over a very short period would not qualify as the illness.

Manic depression has an onset; it is not a disorder that has always been apparent, although it can become a very persistent problem. It is not a personality type but presents as a change or at the very least an exaggeration of the underlying personality. It has a wide range of symptoms so that vastly different faces of the illness can show over time. This means that you can see extraordinary changes in manic depressives that make the person hardly recognisable between one state and another. The illness reflects but wildly exaggerates mood changes that we all experience. Although in the extremes of manic depression it is clear that patients are unwell, there is a graduation back to normal mood that challenges all of us to define what 'normal' is.

1.2 What is bipolar affective disorder?

Psychiatrists may appear to be always changing the names of the illnesses that they treat but this is not always done just to confuse the innocent! Manic depression is a term that has been used for more than a century to cover psychiatric illnesses with the fundamental symptom of a mood change. Fifty years ago the term would have been used widely to cover not only those patients who had manic episodes but also to include those who only experienced severe depression. In the 1960s it became apparent that there are major differences between those patients that experience mania and those that only suffer from depression. The differences are particularly in the course and the family history of the two types of mood illness. However, the considerable overlap has always been recognised. In order to indicate the separation, two new terms were adopted: unipolar and bipolar – unipolar depression for those patients that only experience depression and bipolar affective disorder for those that experience mania (and usually also depression). It would make logical sense to also have a unipolar mania category but in fact the unipolar manics are so similar to the bipolars that this term has not been popular (*see Q 1.13*).

Manic depression is an unusual illness in that a number of people have a bipolar illness that is currently undiagnosed because so far they have only suffered from depression. Even though the illness might have started with depression in the teenage years it is only when mania appears in the twenties that the diagnosis can be made. The illness affects both genders in essentially the same way.

The terms bipolar disorder and manic depression are now commonly used to describe the same illness and this book will follow that practice.

1.3   What do you call recurrent depression with hypomania?

The dividing line between mania and hypomania is not easy to demarcate (*see Q 1.7*); however it is worthwhile making this distinction because it affects decisions about treatment (*Fig. 1.1*). For this reason a different name is given to depression with mania – bipolar I – in contrast to depression with hypomania – bipolar II. There have been attempts to define bipolar III and IV based on family history and the effect of antidepressants but these have not really caught on.

1.4   What are the symptoms of mania?

The following example of a manic woman illustrates the range of symptoms and behaviours characteristic of mania (*see also Box 1.1*).

■ *Mood:* In order to make a diagnosis of mania there must be a change in mood. This is usually elevated and she feels elated, 'great', 'fantastic'.

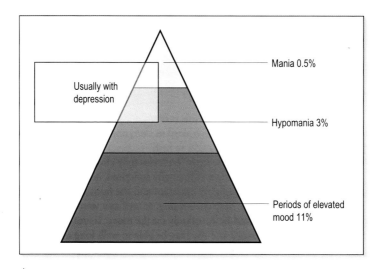

Fig. 1.1 Prevalence of manic depression. (Reprinted from *Clin Appr Bipolar Disord* 2002;1:10–14 by permission of Cambridge Medical Publications.)

BOX 1.1 The symptoms of mania

There must be a change in mood – elation or irritability – together with usually all of the following:
- decreased need for sleep
- increased energy and activity
- excessive talk, with pressure of speech and flight of ideas (*see Box 1.2*)
- fast thoughts
- distractibility and disinhibition (in speech, thoughts and action)
- excessive confidence leading to grandiosity.

Extreme terms are used to describe a state that few of us reach. She may well be feeling 'better than ever', and in an exciting and unique way 'connected with the whole world'. It is common to have never had such a good feeling in the whole of her life. One of the major problems later can be that she doesn't feel that this is an experience that she would like to avoid; in fact she feels just the opposite because it is a feeling that one would want to seek out. The closest comparison is to feelings that a great success or achievement (or winning the lottery) can produce or the high that comes from drugs such as cocaine. The elation is often infectious and others can (at first at least) feel more cheerful in her presence and find a smile on their face. She looks happy but in an active, excited way rather than displaying a calm peaceful serenity.

However, not uncommonly it is irritability rather than elation that is felt and apparent to others. She can't tolerate any disagreement but finds arguments everywhere, as her plans are being thwarted by others who see how unrealistic they are.

- *Sleep:* Sleep is reduced, but this is often not perceived as a problem but rather 'I don't need as much sleep as everyone else – and there is too much to do to spend all night in bed!'

- *Energy:* Energy levels are high: 'batteries fully charged and switched on'. She feels physically and mentally energised, active and strong. Overactivity is immediately apparent and she finds sitting for more than a few minutes very challenging, as well as a waste of time. She may run, dance and be constantly on the move. Increased energy also improves endurance and she may be able to walk long distances without getting tired and ignore the pain of walking barefoot.

- *Attention span:* Attention can be intense but only for a short period. Concentration is poor because of distractibility, so that she cannot spend more than a few minutes on any task before setting off on another track. Memory is perceived to be good but may actually be poor because of the distraction and lack of focus. Afterwards she may have very poor recall of the events during the spell of mania.

■ *Ideas and thoughts:* These flow quickly, freely and fast; speech reflects this. The content is cheerful, confident and inventive until irritability and annoyance take over.

■ *Self-belief:* Overconfidence is the norm and this grows to grandiosity, claiming superior talents and achievements. Her self-belief may be very persuasive to those that don't know her; some may go along with her plans initially, pleased to have found someone with such confidence in themselves, only to be very disappointed later. Grandiosity can become delusional with ideas of royal connections, riches, fame and natural gifts to the extent of superhuman powers (e.g. having control over the weather or ability to predict the future). Arrogance accompanies this, dismissing the views of others (unless they happen to coincide) in a haughty way. Some feel their intellectual powers are high and superior to others and start to talk in a foreign language even though their grasp of grammar and vocabulary may be limited. Physical limitations or disabilities are dismissed – 'I've cured myself of that diabetes' – or minimised or even perceived as signs of superiority. Mental wellbeing is reflected in a sense of physical wellbeing.

■ *Speech:* She will talk non-stop and be difficult to interrupt. Staying quiet becomes impossible and dialogue is not needed – monologue is fine. In fact she does not even need an audience: you can see her wandering about, chatting away. Talking may not be enough – singing, shouting and laughter all form part of expressing her joy to the world.

Flight of ideas is the classic form of speech in mania (*Box 1.2*). Flight indicates the way ideas flow from one to another. The connections within the speech are usually apparent, in contrast to the thought disorder of schizophrenia which is much more obscure. But connections are too free and frequent so that distractions in what she sees or hears send her off on a new track. Alternatively, internal connections or personal memories may suddenly intervene. Playing with language is common as punning or rhyming takes over the flow for a while. The digressions mean that the goals of speech are quickly lost and so little is achieved in any conversation.

BOX 1.2 Flight of ideas

'People are cleaning up the house, working very hard, there's Flash on the floor, the dog doesn't like Flash, there's a flash in my eye as I'm looking at the trees, there's not much oxygen from the trees, there's water on the floor, *agua* run the water, don't block the sink.'

■ *Appetite:* Appetite may be little changed though she will lose weight because essentials such as eating are not given much priority, or poor concentration and distractibility leave everything half eaten.

■ *Disinhibition:* You may notice the disinhibition from a distance with flamboyant, bright, eccentric clothes and a home visit reveals a spectacularly decorated house. It is always interesting to visit a house in the summer which is decked out for Christmas because 'I'm the second coming'. However, be wary of the conservatively dressed Englishman whose dress belies his extraordinary behaviour.

The manic patient may do what the rest of us only think of – she may swear at the boss or alternatively tell him she's in love with him, or head off to Paris on a whim with no bags required. However, involvement in areas which have a high potential for trouble – drinking, taking drugs, overspending and having sex – can be enjoyed at the time but are a source of shame on recovery.

■ *Later stages:* The fun of mania rarely lasts long and the initial infectious cheerfulness degenerates into unstoppable destructive irresponsibility. Others trying to bring her back to earth are dismissed, abused and ignored as the bank account gets emptied and exploiters strip her of her assets and dignity. Her ideas become obviously farcical and she becomes a figure of pity if not ridicule. Finally, someone takes action to get her behaviour curtailed and the indignity of the Mental Health Act assessment, with police backup to take her off to hospital as she will not recognise the extent of her illness, becomes the inevitable consequence. Lack of insight is the classic feature of madness and is to be expected in mania.

1.5 What psychotic symptoms accompany mania?

Psychosis is usually only found in the more extreme states of mania when the other symptoms are prominent. Psychosis refers to distortions of reality up to the point of losing contact with reality. The usual way to recognise psychosis is by the presence of delusions and hallucinations. However, sometimes activity is so bizarre (e.g. someone charging round a building site pretending to do battle training) that it is clear that reality testing is poor.

In mania, delusions are more common than hallucinations; both usually have a grandiose flavour and often come together. It can be difficult to tell when grandiose ideas tip over into delusions. When does thinking you are a good musician become so extreme an idea that it is delusional? The border is when the idea is fixed and is not retracted through logical argument. Some grandiose ideas are so eccentric that they are obviously delusional (e.g. the man claiming to be the Martian ambassador) and don't need testing by argument. Challenging grandiose delusions can easily bring out irritability, if you are not just simply dismissed.

Paranoid ideas are the other type of delusion that is commonly seen in manic states. However, it can be difficult to tell when patients' frustration with others' lack of enthusiasm for their projects turns to paranoia. Paranoia always has a grandiose edge to it: 'Why on earth would the CIA be interested in following you?' Sometimes the mixture is more interesting – for example the man who has to leave the hospital as he is the only one who can tackle the drug traffickers who are in turn out to kill him. But remember paranoid ideas are common in a wide variety of psychiatric disorders (including confusional states) and are certainly not diagnostic of mania.

Hallucinations are most commonly auditory and usually second person ('You're the greatest'), rather than third person ('Look at him, he's so handsome') which is more characteristic of schizophrenia. However, just because certain types of hallucination are present you should not dismiss the diagnosis of mania: so-called 'first rank symptoms of schizophrenia' are common in severe mania.

Visions can occur but are often overinterpretations of 'fantastic sights' – for example a beautiful star-filled night sky is reported as a 'choir of angels'.

Psychotic symptoms in mania are usually mood congruent, i.e. they reflect the underlying mood, either of elation or of irritability, rather than being disconnected and bizarre.

Confusion and visual hallucinations should prompt consideration of a possible organic (or drug-related) state but confusion can occur particularly in postpartum states.

1.6 How much do people remember of their mania afterwards?

It is often surprising how situations that are burnt into the doctor's mind because of the drama are dismissed rather lightly by patients afterwards. This is not universal, and certainly sexual indiscretions can weigh heavily on people afterwards. However, many bipolars have a very poor memory of their mania which can make collecting a retrospective history difficult. Even if you specifically ask about manic symptoms you may get a denial, unless you can discuss the specifics of their behaviour. Patients may also refer to these periods as depression, often because they do remember the depression that followed.

This poor recall can be a blessing for some but can also lead to patients not taking their problem very seriously when it comes to considering preventive treatment.

1.7 What is hypomania?

As the name suggests (Greek, *hypo*, under), hypomania is the same condition as mania but with a lesser degree of symptoms and more importantly less impairment and disability. In fact hypomania can be a very desirable state, with the patient feeling very well physically and mentally, having lots of energy, not needing much sleep, thinking fast with lots of ideas and feeling confident. Although there may be lots of ideas, productivity is often low: 'I've got all the ideas but I can't put anything into practice'. However, unlike mania, concentration can still be good and psychotic symptoms are not present.

The border between hypomania and mania is not clear and there are a number of different definitions. The most useful definition draws a clinical line so that if the symptoms are causing clear disability and last more than a few (e.g. 4) days, then this is mania. If symptoms are below that line then it is hypomania.

As you would expect, it is unusual for patients to present to doctors with hypomania, as it would not be seen as a condition requiring treatment even if they do recognise the change from their normal state. However, many (but not all) people who experience hypomania also have periods of depression which they find distressing and disabling.

Why do so many psychiatrists call patients hypomanic when they are clearly at an extreme of mental illness with manic symptoms? It may be that the term 'manic' is seen as rather derogatory and 'hypomanic' seems less worrying and extreme. Many of us hang on to the way we used terms when we were training and minding our language is a challenge for all of us!

1.8 What are the symptoms of depression?

As for mania, the basic symptom of depression has to be a change of mood. The mood is usually described as sad, unhappy, down or even just 'depressed'. The common feature is that it is a dysphoric and unpleasant mood change. Some patients experience prominent anxiety rather than feeling down; others are very irritable (*Box 1.3*).

BOX 1.3 The symptoms of depression

There is a dysphoric change in mood – sad, miserable, depressed (and often irritable) – together with:
- decreased ability to sleep
- decreased energy and activity leading to retardation
- reduced speech
- sluggish thinking
- poor concentration and memory
- negative thinking – a disparaging view of self and the present situation, and a pessimistic view of the future, along with suicidal thoughts.

■ *Energy:* Energy is low – 'the switch has been turned off'. The depressed feel tired all the time; even minor tasks can seem too much and some will spend the whole day in bed doing nothing. The lack of energy may be obvious to others as they see the patient just sit apparently doing nothing and sometimes hardly even moving. Speech can be very slow with long gaps and the patient seems to take an age to answer a simple question. This does seem to be an actual slowing of the thought processes and patients do come to the right answer if you wait long enough. Others may be very agitated, pacing around wringing their hands, sighing, not able to sit down and endlessly restless, not knowing what to do with themselves.

■ *Memory and concentration:* Memory is decreased, sometimes to the point that patients think they must be starting to dement because they cannot remember straightforward things like the name of a friend or what they have gone into the garage to get – though all of us experience this at times! This is at least partly due to concentration being poor. This can be a lack of attention – for example when reading, although the words on the page go in, they are not registered, and the patient cannot give an account of the content.

■ *Negative thoughts:* The world of the depressed is focused internally which can prevent events outside being either recognised or given much importance. Many of the depressed are distracted by their own unpleasant thoughts going round and round so that the only things they can concentrate on are the negative ideas that are dominating thinking. When depressed there is a strong negative bias to all the thinking processes. Unpleasant memories are much more easily recalled than pleasant ones, so that a patient may be unable to recall anything nice that has happened this year, whereas even apparently minor adversities are readily called to mind.

Depressives will almost certainly see themselves as worthless, useless and not worth bothering with – arguing with close family who are trying to get them to see how much they are valued. They see the world as an unpleasant hostile place that offers little solace. As Hardy wrote: 'Happiness was but the occasional episode in a general drama of pain.' Many depressives would have trouble even noticing the occasional episode of happiness. Their negativity can be quite infectious and the depressed can make others feel uncomfortable and so lead to them being avoided. The other habit that tends to alienate the depressed is their tendency to reveal a lot of personal details while portraying themselves very negatively.

■ *Suicide:* A negative view of the future is one of the drivers to suicide. The negative bias includes feelings that nothing can change and only bad things can happen from now on, and of only being a burden to loved ones. It is easy to see how, for a depressive, there is only a small step to thinking: 'Everyone would be better off without me and I would be out of this mental pain if I was dead.' Thinking about death is almost universal in depression and suicidal thoughts from 'I sometimes just wish I wouldn't wake up in the morning' through to clear ideas of self-harm should be expected.

■ *Physical manifestations:* Some people have prominent physical symptoms when depressed, often exacerbations of prior physical problems such as worsening backache, as they become more sensitive to pain. Others will develop new physical symptoms such as headaches and other tension symptoms or stomach pains, or just feel generally unwell and tired. Depressed patients are likely to worry about these physical symptoms and what they mean, such as thinking that they must have cancer to explain the feeling in the stomach, nausea and weight loss, or that poor memory means dementia is on the horizon.

■ *Appetite:* Loss of appetite and consequently losing weight is the rule, although a few patients report an increase in appetite – often favouring sweet foods.

■ *Sleep:* Sleep problems usually occur and it is unusual to find a depressed patient who is sleeping well. The classic symptom is early morning waking when the patient wakes up, feeling bad and completely unable to get back to sleep or even to relax in bed and rest, despite feeling exhausted. However, initial insomnia is common, when the patient goes to bed tired but suddenly finds that sleep is elusive. Waking frequently during the night is also a common complaint. In fact we all wake a few times at night but don't remember it because it is brief, but the depressed will wake and then stay awake, possibly because worry sets in. Nightmares are common and the pleasant release of dreams is rare. Some patients will oversleep and spend not only the night but much of the day in bed and asleep, feeling too tired to raise themselves.

1.9 What psychotic symptoms occur in bipolar depression?

Delusional ideas are congruent with the depressed mood, i.e. the content of delusions is very negative – 'My insides are rotting'. Depressives can feel so guilty that they think that they must have committed a terrible crime and need to be punished. It is unusual for the more bizarre delusions seen in schizophrenia to be present and the relationship of the delusion to the mood is usually obvious. Psychotic symptoms are usually only present when the other symptoms of depression are very obvious and severe: it is worth considering if the diagnosis is correct if psychosis is evident but only mild physical symptoms of depression are found.

Hallucinations are usually auditory, i.e. hearing a voice saying nasty things – for example hearing children in a playground shouting

'Paedophile!', or a voice saying 'You're going to burn in Hell'. Although other modalities of hallucination occur – for example smelling the body rotting – these are uncommon.

1.10 In what way are the symptoms of depression in bipolars different from those of unipolars?

The symptoms are very similar in bipolar and unipolar depression and any differences are not consistent. Bipolars are more likely to show excessive sleep and more lability of mood; they are also more subject to psychotic symptoms. Other common features are abrupt onset and sudden recovery.

The course of bipolar illness tends to be that patients have their first episode at a younger age and they are more likely to experience frequent recurrences. As a group, bipolars are more likely to have a family history of depression and also of bipolar disorder. However, even taking all these factors into account it is really not possible to tell when seeing a depressed patient if they are bipolar or likely to become bipolar. It can be surprising when patients whom you know well and have treated for depression suddenly become manic for the first time.

1.11 What is a mixed affective state?

The usual view of manic depression is of the two extremes of mood – very high and very low – which are seen as opposites. However, there is more in common between these states than it at first appears. Both states involve loss of sleep; overactivity is obvious in mania but it can also be present in depression in the form of agitation. The rushing thoughts of mania are apparent in speech but in depression the mind is often full of overwhelming negative thoughts going round and round that cannot be stopped. Both mood states lead to poor concentration, memory and distractibility. Psychosis can be evident in both states, though usually in different forms; disability is profound in both states when severe.

It is easier to understand 'switching' when the similarities between the two states are appreciated. Many depressions are followed by mania and vice versa. This is often put down to the effect of the medication but in fact it is a basic part of the illness course and was apparent well before the treatments we currently use were available.

It is probably better to look on mania and depression as closely related states rather than opposites and that they have more in common with each other than with euthymia (Greek, *eu*, good; *thymia*, mood) – normal mood (*Fig. 1.2A*). This makes the understanding of mixed states easier and the more you look for mixed states the more you will see them.

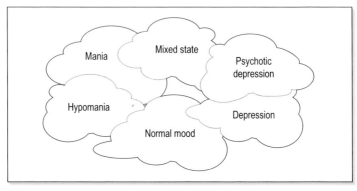

A

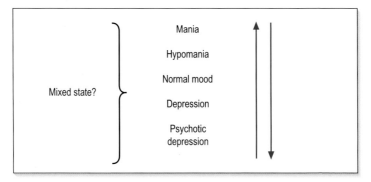

B

▲

Fig. 1.2 A, The relationship of mania and depression to normal mood. **B,** Depression and mania are not best seen as opposite states.

Mixed states are the combination of manic and depressive symptoms at the same time (*Fig. 1.2B*). Sometimes it is just the presence of depressive ideas: feeling guilty and frightened in an otherwise clear manic state – dysphoric mania (*Case vignette 1.1*). For others the combination is so marked that you cannot say in which state they are in:

■ Is this overactivity or agitation?
■ Why is he looking so cheerful but talking about the world dying?
■ You are quietly discussing her suicidal thoughts when she laughs at you and makes a silly pun.

■ In the morning he can hardly get out of bed but by the evening he's joking with his children and making wild plans to redecorate the house only to slump back that night.

The treatment of mood disorders requires you to make a judgement about the predominant mood state to focus treatment. However, if you are in serious doubt or the condition is clearly a mixed state, then the right approach is to treat as you would mania. Mixed states are usually less responsive to treatments and it is advisable to aim for some longer term treatment that is likely to prevent relapse rather than focus just on the current episode. Valproate is likely to be more effective than lithium in treating a mixed state.

A good general approach in bipolar illness is to focus on long-term considerations rather than just on the current symptoms. Looking only at the immediately apparent symptoms can lead to making frequent changes in treatment to deal with a changing clinical picture whereas enhancing the long-term treatment is more likely to lead to sustained improvements in stability and mood.

CASE VIGNETTE 1.1 MIXED AFFECTIVE STATE

Susan breezes into the consulting room, saying: 'I haven't been right doctor'. You expect her to rapidly reel off manic symptoms but instead she says 'I've been very down, worried about my mother – she's ill again, I can't sleep – up all night, can't be right – given them all a fright'. She laughs as she describes the problems her mother's decline into dementia are causing everyone. She looks cheerful but what she is saying does not match at all her apparent high spirits. She then bursts into tears: 'You'll have to shrink and wrap me back up again'. Her speech is disordered, playing with words and very distractible, but is she manic or depressed? She is in a mixed state.

1.12 What does rapid cycling mean?

The frequency of recurrence in manic depression is very variable. The usual pattern is an episodic illness with a sustained recovery for several months or even years between episodes. Many will have an individual episode which consists of a period of both depression and mania which follow straight on from one another and then recovery ensues.

However, some patients have a very unstable illness which is frequently changing. Rapid cycling is usually defined as having four episodes in 1 year; this could mean alternating between mania and depression twice in a year or having episodes separated by periods of being in normal mood. The pattern is so variable that one person's rapid cycling can be very different from that of another. Someone may have six episodes of depression in a year, each lasting a few weeks but then recovery in between; another patient can be ill throughout the year but move several times between mania and depression. The speed of changing between episodes can become very fast so that week to week the patient is in a different phase of the illness and sometimes it becomes so extreme that the illness changes from one day to the next. At this extreme it can be difficult to disentangle from a mixed affective state when people have facets of both mania and depression in the same day (*see Q 6.23*).

Rapid cycling is uncommon and at any one time fewer than 5% of manic depressives will be in this state. It is more common among those who are taking antidepressant drugs; stopping these is the first line of treatment and can make a dramatic difference to the course of the illness. It is also worth checking thyroid function as this is commonly associated with unstable bipolar illness.

Rapid cycling does tend to resolve itself in the longer run, and it is unusual to stay in this state for more than a year.

Treatment approaches for rapid cycling that can be helpful include stopping antidepressants and a change in long-term treatment: for example valproate may prove more effective than lithium for rapid cyclers. However, this may just be a statement of the obvious as if a patient is on lithium and becomes a rapid cycler then lithium is clearly not working well. It may also be true that if a patient is on valproate and develops rapid cycling then lithium may prove to be more effective.

1.13 Why do we not have a condition called unipolar mania?

Some people do define unipolar mania as a patient who has experienced at least three episodes of mania but no serious depression. However, the point of making a more specific diagnosis is to indicate either a biologically different condition or a different prognosis. Neither of these seems to apply as if you compare unipolar manics with bipolars you find no difference in the age of onset of the illness, how frequently they relapse, their response to treatment or their family history. As you would expect, follow-up of the unipolar manics shows that at least a third will have to be reclassified as bipolar when they finally develop a depression.

1.14 Do bipolars suffer from other psychiatric problems?

Unfortunately (but not unexpectedly) this is true and watching out for comorbid problems is an important task in the medical care of these patients. Substance misuse is the most common additional disorder, and there are high rates of all the common addictions (smoking, alcohol and illicit drugs), as well as twice the rates of

> unipolar depression which are themselves nearly twice those of the general population. Anxiety disorders afflict a quarter of manic depressives and are easy to miss as many patients see these as aspects of their personality that would not be worthy of consultation in their own right.

Sometimes anxiety is a part of the depression but it is commonly a problem in its own right when patients have otherwise recovered. It is likely that the anxiety problems make a major contribution to the substance misuse as patients try to damp down their symptoms with alcohol or other drugs.

1.15 What is schizoaffective disorder?

Probably two-thirds of patients with mania have psychotic symptoms (but a smaller proportion of depressions) and often these delusions and hallucinations are similar to the ideas and experiences found in schizophrenia. The main difference between the psychoses of schizophrenia and bipolar disorder is that you would expect the psychotic symptoms to disappear as the manic or depressive symptoms recede. Schizoaffective disorder refers to those patients whose psychosis does not fit this neat pattern of a close relationship between affective and psychotic symptoms.

There is a large number of definitions of schizoaffective disorder and a pragmatic approach to these definitions, based on what treatment approach is likely to be most useful, is recommended.

There is a group of patients who suffer from depression but also have prominent psychotic symptoms, both during the depression and outside of periods of depression, who are actually on the border (if not in the territory) of schizophrenia. Some of these people would qualify as schizoaffective. There are many patients who suffer from schizophrenia who also experience (commonly) depression and (occasionally) mania. Usually the depressed schizophrenics would stay in the schizophrenia group but those who become manic would usually be put in a schizoaffective category.

There are also people with clear manic and depressive episodes who, when you saw them in an episode of illness, you would clearly classify as manic depressive. However, when they recover they still have some persistent psychotic symptoms – either delusions or hallucinations – which require treatment in their own right. These people are in the grey area between schizophrenia and manic depression and this is the main group that would be classified as schizoaffective as treatment needs to be focused on both types of symptom (*Fig. 1.3* and Case vignette 6.3).

Antipsychotics are the mainstay of treatment in schizophrenia and schizoaffective disorders, but mood symptoms may also be a target for treatment.

1.16 Why does it take several years for some patients to get a correct diagnosis of bipolar disorder?

When you look back at the history of people with manic depression it is very common to find that it takes up to 10 years for the correct diagnosis to be reached (*Case vignette 1.2*). This can be for the practical reason that they were only suffering from depression for several years and so it was not possible to make a bipolar diagnosis until the manic episode appeared!

Many people do suffer from manic symptoms but these are not recognised as such by the patient or the doctor. Usually this is because they are feeling exceptionally well and so do not see the need to consult for this! They may present with depression but they and the doctor are focused on this aspect and so high moods are not discussed. Even if they are asked, it can be very difficult for people to remember high moods during depression. When depressed, memory becomes very selective so that only negative events and emotions are readily recalled.

Manic symptoms can also get buried in alcohol and drug misuse. It is common for those who are manic to drink heavily or to take drugs. The disinhibition and irritability of mania are then put down to the alcohol or drugs and not recognised as symptoms of mania.

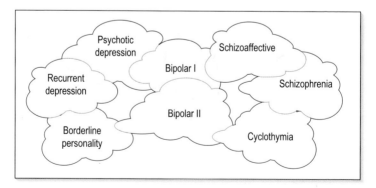

▲

Fig. 1.3 The relationship of bipolar disorder to other psychiatric illnesses.

Many manic episodes are characterised by irritability rather than elation. This is less easy to recognise and more likely to be seen as an aspect of personality rather than as an illness. This can be a particularly difficult problem to unravel but it can be very useful to go through all the symptoms of mania to make as good an assessment as possible.

At the other end of the spectrum young people can present with a severe psychotic illness with disturbed behaviour, again often complicated by drug misuse. The diagnosis can then be unclear as to whether this is mania, schizophrenia or a drug-induced state. It is common for those who have severe manic depression to be given an early diagnosis of acute schizophrenia. If you see this in the notes but are sure the current symptoms are manic then you are probably right. In the acute situation this may not make much difference to the treatment but it will make a difference to estimating prognosis and deciding long-term treatment.

CASE VIGNETTE 1.2 REACHING THE CORRECT DIAGNOSIS

Liz was referred but her husband attended as she would not come. In fact she had left home and rented a flat in Birmingham where she had some friends. He described a usually confident woman who had a wide circle of friends gradually changing over the last year. She seemed more irritable and dissatisfied and they had been getting into a lot of arguments. They had stopped sleeping together as she seemed to have become very restless at night and disturbed him.

Over the past 2 weeks their relationship had deteriorated and she had left. He had tried to stop her driving away and she had bumped the car into the wall trying to avoid him. She had been arrested later that evening because she was speeding and had initially failed an alcohol breath test but was later released.

Two months later she did come to the clinic. She was depressed and feeling terrible, she still did not think that all the previous martial problems were entirely her fault but did accept that she had been behaving erratically. She had spent 6 weeks in Birmingham, had enjoyed some of this and spent a lot of money. Her friends had been very welcoming at first and took her side against her husband but they gradually got fed up with her and encouraged her to go back home. By this time her mood was changing and she felt that she could not cope living on her own.

She described several periods of depression over the previous 15 years for which she had not sought treatment. She had also suffered a breakdown in her teens which led to her spending 2 months in hospital. She had hated this experience, blamed her mother for it and it had made her very averse to seeing doctors.

She did not think that she suffered from manic depression, but over the following 2 years did agree to try treatment with lithium and was pleasantly surprised to find that she went through a whole year without a period of depression.

1.17 How can I improve my ability to diagnose bipolar disorder?

You will be able to find patients that you can clearly classify: those with unipolar recurrent depressions and other patients with a clear manic depressive illness. However, there are a large number of patients in the middle who are much more challenging diagnostically. The two main problems in making the diagnosis are eliciting the symptoms and making a judgement.

ELICITING THE SYMPTOMS

This is a particular problem when a patient is depressed and does not recall periods of elation as memory bias is so negative: even if you have asked the right questions you have not got the right information.

Despite these problems it is worth asking all those who suffer from depression a non-specific question such as: 'Have there been times when you've had the opposite problem to depression; been too high and excited?' There are some screening questionnaires that can be used and although their discriminatory rate is not good, they do give some examples of useful questions (see Hirschfeld 2000, www.bipolar.com/mdq.htm). It can also be useful to ask an informant such as a spouse or parent, though unfortunately quite often you gain contradictory views from informants and patients. The situation can arise where the patient gives what appears to be a clear history of hypomania but then the relative says they have never noticed any of this!

MAKING A JUDGEMENT

When you have the information, you then have the second problem in that you have to make a judgement as to whether this crosses the line between normal variation and hypomania or between hypomania and mania. Even the most expert clinician has difficulty in making these judgements and their meaning in terms of treatment is still under dispute. You should be basing this judgement on the presence of symptoms, their severity, pervasiveness and persistence.

The essence of treatment of these conditions is long-term involvement and, as with many illnesses, it becomes clearer as time goes on, so it is entirely reasonable to shift your diagnosis as you become more familiar with the clinical course. You are much more likely to make serious mistakes if you are too wedded to your diagnosis and therefore unwilling to change when contradictory information arises. (The situation I have been most caught out in is when I have made a diagnosis of personality disorder and drug misuse and then find it difficult to accept when I see evidence of manic and depressive syndromes.)

PATIENT QUESTIONS

1.18 But my mother just isn't a depressed type of person

There is a common misconception that only certain types of people are
liable to depression and manic depression. It is true that there are some
personalities who are 'depressive', by which we mean that they have always
been unhappy people who tend to be pessimistic and see the negative side of
life. These people are also very likely to suffer periods of depression on top
of their usual negativity.

  Most people who suffer from depression as part of a bipolar illness are not
of this personality type and when well you would not recognise them as
being likely to get depressed. This can be quite a hurdle to overcome in
accepting the illness both in members of your family and in yourself. That is
why we consider manic depression to be an illness, i.e. a state that can afflict
almost anyone, and it is not possible to predict who will get the illness.

Causes and course of the illness

2

PQ PATIENT QUESTIONS

CAUSES

2.1   How common is bipolar disorder?

The simplest answer to this is that it occurs in 1% of people. This seems to be true around the world in any population investigated. However, there is a spectrum from severe mania through milder forms of manic depression to recurrent depression and on to normal mood variation. It is always difficult when you have a spectrum to know exactly where to draw the lines within this to define the different disorders. Tight definitions of manic depression would give a figure of less than 1%; broader definitions which include hypomania would give figures from 2 up to 10% (*Fig. 2.1*).

2.2   What causes manic depression?

'Nature or nurture, genes or environment?' is a common question in the cause of any illness that is rarely answered definitively. For bipolar illness (particularly the more severe end of the spectrum – mania rather than hypomania) the genes/nature answer seems more likely. Bipolar illness tends to run in families and the more closely an individual is related by blood to a manic depressive the more likely that person is to develop the illness. If one parent suffers from manic depression and a child is adopted away and brought up by another family, there is still the same risk of developing manic depression as if the child was brought up by the biological parents. In the case of twins, if one twin suffers from manic

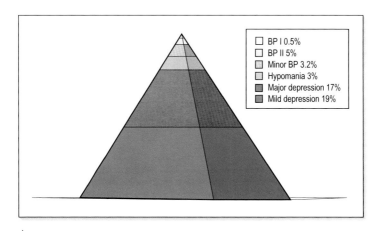

BP I 0.5%
BP II 5%
Minor BP 3.2%
Hypomania 3%
Major depression 17%
Mild depression 19%

Fig. 2.1 The prevalence of affective disorders. BP, bipolar. (Reprinted from *Clin Appr Bipolar Disord* 2002;1:10–14 by permission of Cambridge Medical Publications.)

depression then the chance of the other twin becoming ill is higher in cases of identical rather than fraternal twins (Smoller & Finn 2003). All of these observations indicate that bipolar illness is strongly influenced by genetic factors. However, it is not the whole story as even identical twins are not 100% concordant: if one identical twin suffers from manic depression the other will have a bipolar illness in about 50% of cases and recurrent depression in about 30%. However, there are still 20% of identical twins who are discordant, i.e. one is illness-free.

2.3 What family history am I likely to elicit from a patient with manic depression?

About 70% of bipolar patients will have a close relative (a parent or sibling) who suffers either from manic depression or from serious (usually recurrent) depression. Only 20% will actually have a bipolar relative (*Case vignette 2.1*). The equivalent figures for the general population are about 10% (depression) and 1% (bipolar). First-degree relatives (sibling, parent or child) of someone who is manic depressive have about a 10–15% chance of having or developing manic depression (Gershon et al 1982, Gottesman 1991, Smoller & Finn 2003) (*Fig. 2.2*).

Relatives of bipolar patients do however have a higher chance of being successful academically and occupationally. It is only a small effect but may indicate that having a small dose of what leads to manic depression can actually be an advantage.

CASE VIGNETTE 2.1 FAMILY HISTORY PROVIDES IMPORTANT INFORMATION FOR CLINICAL DECISIONS

James is 47. You already know him as you treated his mother who suffered from manic depression but who died several years ago. You have also treated his son who has a bipolar illness and is now 20 and on a combination of lithium and valproate because his illness was difficult to control. James now presents with symptoms of depression. In particular he is very low in energy and motivation. He is sleeping excessively and although usually a very active, self-employed man, is doing very little at the moment. He has no history of mania or hypomania in the past nor has he ever had a previous episode of depression. The question is, therefore, should James be treated with antidepressants as would any other patient *without* this family history or should he be treated with lithium, either on its own initially or in combination with an antidepressant?

Judgement in this case was to treat James with an antidepressant – an SSRI initially which would reduce the chances of switching into mania. However, he needed to be warned that there was a distinct possibility he might develop a bipolar illness and for him and his family to keep an eye open for symptoms of mania or hypomania. In view of the history, there would be a very low threshold for starting him on a mood stabiliser such as lithium.

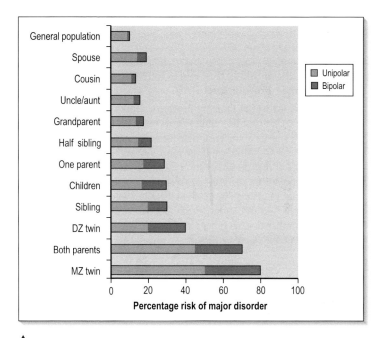

▲

Fig. 2.2 The possible relationship between the closeness of the blood relationship to someone with manic depression and the likelihood of developing depression and bipolar disorder. DZ, dizygotic; MZ, monozygotic.

2.4   How many genes are involved?

It is possible that some families with several members with manic depression have single genes having a major effect, although in most cases it is likely to be several genes that increase the liability to manic depression. These genes are likely to overlap with the genes that predispose to severe and recurrent depression and also with those predisposing to psychosis including schizophrenia. It is probable that we all have some of these genes and that those who suffer the illness have more of the susceptibility genes and in particular combinations. However, despite a major research investment in this area we are not yet at the point of predicting who is particularly susceptible to manic depression from examination of their genes. The other hope from genetic research is that we might be able to identify which patients are likely to respond to which medicines from an analysis of their genes.

The questions that are likely to emerge include: 'What are the normal functions of these genes?' and 'To what extent do we need to be liable to depression and elation?'

2.5 Why are there genes that cause extreme emotions prevalent in the 'normal' population?

One theory is that the ability to develop a depressed mood has been selected for in our recent (last few million years) evolutionary development and is vital to our social competence. The facts that mood disorders tend to be more common in women and the most vulnerable time is in the postnatal period suggest that the ability for a mother to become depressed has some reproductive advantage. How could this be when it would seem a major disadvantage to get depressed when there is a baby to look after? Perhaps depression is best seen as the mental equivalent of pain. How would we expect a mother to react if her baby died? We would of course expect her to become depressed and would be very surprised if she did not. In fact we would not really regard this depression as a psychiatric problem because it would be so understandable. Our evolutionary tactic has been to have a small number of offspring but to take very good care of them, rather than have many and rely on a few surviving. A mechanism that meant mothers would know that their baby dying would lead to extreme mental distress would seem to be a powerful additional factor in ensuring that mothers take very good care of their offspring. Of course, like other pain mechanisms, it can go wrong and activate when not beneficial and this may be what constitutes the depression end of manic depression.

The advantages of hypomania are probably easier to recognise, when increased energy, attention and optimism can still bring results even in (or perhaps particularly in) this modern era. But the extreme of mania could be this mechanism going wrong.

If the genes that are responsible for manic depression are identified, then the next question to be answered is: 'What kind of world would we be living in if we identified and eliminated the genes responsible for manic depression?'

2.6 Which genes cause the illness?

There has been a huge investment in trying to discover the particular genes that relate to manic depression. Many genes have been looked at and several have initially shown promise, but at this point no clear linkage has been established which can be replicated consistently. It seems likely that the problem will prove much more complicated than we had hoped and differences in how genes are expressed may be as important as differences between variations (alleles) of a particular gene.

There is another problem when looking at the genetics of manic depression, i.e. what constitutes manic depression?

■ We would all include those with a bipolar I disorder, but would we also include bipolar II patients?

■ How about those who suffer recurrent depression but have family members with bipolar illness?

■ Would we include all those with recurrent severe depression?

The question of where we draw the lines around the phenotype is still one of the basic questions that need to be answered (*see Ch. 1*).

2.7 Who is likely to develop manic depression?

There are two ways of finding people who are likely to develop a bipolar illness. The first is looking in the families of those who already suffer from manic depression, as the risks are elevated in close family members (*see Q 2.3*). The second way is to look amongst those who are suffering from depression but have not had episodes of mania. About 15% of those who suffer from recurrent depression will develop mania.

It is not possible to predict who will develop manic depression and it is a continual surprise when those people who have been treated for depression for several years suddenly become manic (*see Case vignette 4.1*). However, those whose illness started at a young age (particularly in the teenage years or the twenties) and those who have frequent episodes and rapid shifts between depression and euthymia are particularly at risk (*Fig. 2.3*).

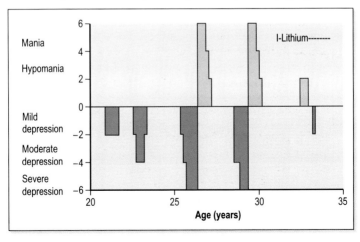

▲

Fig. 2.3 Recurrent depression can precede bipolar disorder.

2.8 Does adversity bring on manic depression or cause relapses?

There is a general assumption when looking at psychiatric disorders that they have been set off by something that has happened in the patient's life. The same assumptions are sometimes made about physical illnesses such as heart attacks and strokes. Working out to what extent this is true is difficult because bad things happen quite often (e.g. we all suffer bereavements) and if an illness occurs it may coincide with an adverse event.

The situation is made more complicated by the fact that we can make bad things happen to us – for example if a husband is abusive to his wife then she may leave. Depression and mania can lead to changes in behaviour which trigger off adverse events. Getting a court summons for speeding may be related to the early symptoms of mania.

There have been several studies (e.g. Hunt et al 1992) that have tried to tease out these various factors which have led to the conclusion that adverse events do play a part. The first episode of manic depression is likely to be at a time of other difficulties in the person's life, and recurrences are also likely to coincide with adverse life events (*Fig. 2.4*). However, the contribution from life events is small and it is best to look at them as triggers rather than causes.

2.9 Does upbringing affect the chance of developing manic depression?

Those who have had a difficult and abusive childhood are more likely to suffer from depression and personality problems. An unhappy childhood

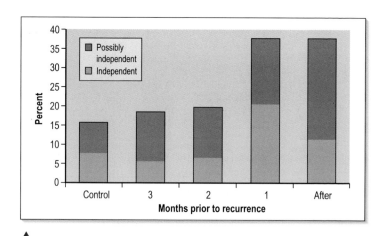

▲

Fig. 2.4 Life events prior to relapses in manic depression.

does not make anyone more liable to develop manic depression and the childhoods of manic depressives are usually normal. Those who suffer from schizophrenia are more likely to have had adverse physical problems in childhood, difficult births with obstetric complications and illnesses such as meningitis, encephalitis and head injury. However, this does not seem to be true for manic depressives – or at least not to the same extent. It is unlikely that adverse childhood experiences offer an explanation for the development of manic depression.

2.10   Are there physical illnesses that can lead to manic depression?

Several organic diseases have been linked with manic depression, particularly in those whose illness begins in older age (over 65). Cerebrovascular disease is the most common; non-dominant hemisphere cerebrovascular accidents in particular appear to predispose to the development of mania but this is still a rare outcome and often there is either a previous history of depression or a family history of affective disorder.

Other brain disorders (or systemic diseases with cerebral involvement) can present with mania or severe (often psychotic) depression. This includes infection with HIV, usually when it reaches the immunodeficiency stage, autoimmune disorders such as systemic lupus erythematosus (SLE) or primary neurological diseases such as multiple sclerosis. Accompanying the affective syndrome there is usually evidence of disorientation and other features of confusion along with visual hallucinations, both of which are uncommon in primary bipolar illness.

> It is clear that thyroid disease can alter the course of manic depression but it may be that it also has a causal association in some people. Abnormalities of other endocrine systems can cause depression and rarely mania, in particular Cushing's disease, where the level of corticosteroids is raised.
>
> It is important to be aware of physical illnesses that can be associated with bipolar disorder and particularly to ensure that thyroid disorder is recognised and treated at an early stage.

2.11   Does the use of illicit drugs cause manic depression?

Stimulant illicit drugs such as amfetamines, cocaine and ecstasy can certainly mimic mania. People who are acutely intoxicated with stimulants usually appear overcheerful, excited, overactive and talkative. Sometimes they will also have paranoid ideas and they usually have difficulty sleeping (or don't want to sleep). The distinguishing features are the history of ingestion, very acute onset and rapid recovery, usually within 24–48 hours.

Stimulant drugs can also precipitate mania among manic depressives. Illicit drugs seriously worsen the course of the illness and its treatment, and invariably the frequency of recurrence, complications and compliance are affected. Whether taking stimulants can actually set off a lifelong propensity to mania and depression is much less certain. If this were beyond doubt, the incidence of manic depression would have increased considerably in recent years and that probably is not the case.

Stimulant drugs can also lead to more persistent depression (up to a few weeks) in the period after prolonged drug use.

Cannabis is associated with the development of psychosis, particularly among heavy users, and is an important causal factor in schizophrenia. Whether it can also induce manic depression is less clear, but it is likely to lead to psychosis, particularly during periods of mania.

2.12 Do any medicines cause mania or depression?

The drugs most often associated with mania are the corticosteroids which ties in with the link with Cushing's disease (*see Q 2.10*). Minor elevations of mood with euphoria are felt by many people taking steroids but it is rare that this extends to the full manic syndrome. However, depression is a more common and debilitating outcome of this treatment.

Those with Parkinson's disease who are having treatment with L-dopa can also experience elevation of mood and other manic symptoms. The use of stimulants including methylphenidate can cause mania (*see Q 2.11*) and this can cause significant problems when considering the diagnosis in adolescents who already have deficits in attention. However, the most common drugs to induce mania are antidepressants (*see Q 3.15*).

There is a long list of drugs that are associated with depression apart from steroids (*Box 2.1*). The induction of depression by the antihypertensive reserpine – which depletes monoamines including noradrenaline (norepinephrine) and serotonin – was the original basis for the theory that monoamines were the important neurotransmitters in depression.

2.13 Is bipolar illness more common among some ethnic groups?

Manic depression is an illness that is found throughout the world in all countries and cultures. The incidence of the severe end of bipolar illness is similar in different countries, but it is not clear if this is true at the bipolar II end of the spectrum. Surveys looking at rates of hypomania have been undertaken only in developed countries, and the reliability of this diagnosis in surveys is not good.

Several studies show that minority ethnic groups are more likely to develop manic depression. This may be because migrants are particularly vulnerable to this illness, with an increased rate among those who have

> **BOX 2.1 Drugs commonly associated with depression**
>
> ■ Steroids, including prednisolone and dexamethasone
> ■ Beta-blockers, particularly those that cross the blood–brain barrier, including propranolol
> ■ Reserpine
> ■ Oral contraceptives
> ■ Mefloquine
>
> Depression is commonly precipitated in those who are predisposed (especially those with previous episodes).

moved between countries. The explanation for this could be that those who do move have a particular type of personality (energetic, highly motivated, 'hyperthymic') or that the stress of migrating and adapting to a new culture is causal.

2.14 Does a particular personality predispose to bipolar illness?

Personality is a notoriously difficult concept to tie down and the relationship between personality type and manic depression is even more complicated. Traditionally it is the cyclothymic temperament that is associated with bipolar illness. Cyclothymia shows itself as mood swings, both up and down, usually with other symptoms of mania and depression but at a low and subclinical level. We are probably all familiar with someone who shows this, though often they are not very aware of it themselves. Some weeks they are cheerful and sociable and others rather grumpy and miserable – this is true of many of us but particularly true of cyclothymics!

Some people who develop clear manic depression do report cyclothymia as the type of personality that they have had since their teenage years. However, this is uncommon and most people with manic depression would have been considered to have a personality within the realm considered normal prior to their illness developing.

Between episodes of illness, manic depressives revert to their usual personality. This is in quite marked contrast to those who suffer from schizophrenia who often have change in their personality with a blunting of emotional responses.

2.15 Is manic depression becoming more common?

The answer is probably not but we are getting better at recognising the range of manic depressive illnesses (although some would say we have got worse at drawing limits around a serious illness). The closer that epidemiological studies come to looking at the community, rather than judging the prevalence of manic depression from hospital samples, the larger the number of cases that are found. More patients who had previously been treated as suffering from recurrent depression are now recognised as bipolar because, when examined over a long period of time, it is clear they have periods of elevated mood between their episodes of depression.

Some believe that manic depression really is becoming more common, not just better recognised, particularly among those that misuse drugs such as cocaine and anabolic steroids. It may be that this increase is not really a rise in the prevalence of manic depression but an increase in drug-induced manias, as the long-term outcome for these people is not clear.

COURSE

2.16 At what age does manic depression start?

> The first episode can occur at any age after puberty. (Whether episodes of mania occur before puberty is controversial; if it does happen, it is very rare.) The average age is about 30 years but this covers a very broad range (*see Fig. 2.5*). Most patients will have had their first major episode of affective illness in their twenties.

Sometimes patients will recall earlier but more minor episodes going back to their teens. Later onsets are, however, not uncommon, particularly in people who have already experienced depressions. In the elderly mania is much more likely to be preceded in earlier life by periods of depression, so it may not be apparent that this is a bipolar illness until old age. A first episode of mania can certainly occur in the elderly but if there have been no previous periods of depression then physical illness should be excluded as a trigger factor (*see Q 2.10*).

What is striking is that there is usually a gap of 5–10 years between the onset of symptoms and the diagnosis being made (*see Q 1.16*). This is partly because it is impossible to make a bipolar diagnosis when only depression has occurred so far and also because the symptoms of both mania and depression may initially be mild and difficult to recognise. It is also hard to disentangle bipolar symptoms from personality and situational factors in the early years. It can be difficult to make this diagnosis, but it should be borne in mind in everyone who presents with depression. However, this needs to be balanced with falling into the other trap of making the diagnosis when it is not appropriate.

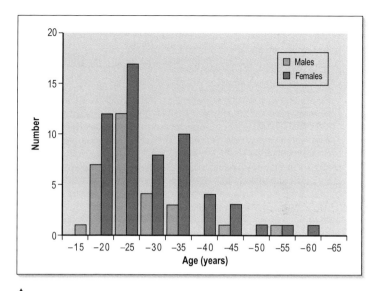

▲

Fig. 2.5 Age of first episode of bipolar disorder.

The earlier the diagnosis can be made, the earlier effective treatment can be provided, thus reducing the impact on the patient's life and improving the long-term outcome.

2.17 Does an early onset mean a more severe condition?

Many people who suffer from manic depression actually date the onset to their teenage years. However they report that the illness is mild during that time and they manage to continue their lives without major disruption. It is only later in life that the episodes become more severe and disabling and they require treatment.

Severe and psychotic episodes can begin at any age including adolescence. Likewise illnesses that do not respond well to treatment and become either chronic or with frequent relapses can occur at any age. Overall the range of severity of the illness and the frequency of relapse are not higher in those with an earlier onset.

The treatment of adolescents with bipolar illness can be very challenging, not intrinsically because of the nature of the illness but because of the nature of the teenager. Teenagers are more likely to have complications such as drug misuse and poor compliance with treatment (*see* Q 6.20)

2.18 How common is recurrence after a single episode of mania?

Recurrence of bipolar disorder is almost inevitable. Single episodes of mania with no further illnesses occur in only 5% of patients. However the gap between illnesses can be many years (*Fig. 2.6*). Recurrence of mania and occurrence of depression are equally likely after recovery from mania.

In the year after a first manic episode about 50% will have an episode of depression or mania. If there have been previous depressions then the risk is even higher. There are really no other factors at first episode that can help predict whether any patient will be particularly likely to experience an early recurrence.

2.19 How long do episodes of mania and depression last?

Looking back at the data collected a hundred years ago it is apparent that most patients did recover in the long run but mania and depression regularly lasted for many months. Modern treatments have meant that most patients will be recovering within a few weeks, with episodes lasting longer being considered 'treatment resistant'.

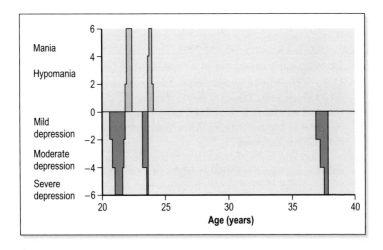

▲

Fig. 2.6 The course of manic depression can include lengthy well intervals. This graph demonstrates a long well interval after four episodes.

2.20 Do patients make a full recovery from each episode?

If this is the first episode of mania or an early episode of depression you can be fairly confident that the patient will recover in that the symptoms will go away entirely. In the early years of suffering from manic depression symptomatic recovery is the norm; however getting back to full function is much harder and there is a fallout in terms of occupational capacity from early on, partly because it is difficult for patients to get back to highly responsible jobs if they have acted very erratically either in mania or in depression (e.g. losing their license to drive a heavy goods vehicle). It is also hard for patients to return to high stress jobs with long hours if they are trying to take good care of their mental and physical health.

2.21 Is it mania or depression which predominates in the long run?

Almost all bipolar patients experience both depression and mania. Women tend to have an illness course that is predominantly depressive, men tend to have more manic spells and fewer depressions. Unipolar mania is sometimes defined as having three episodes of mania and none of depression, and this is more commonly found among men.

For any individual patient the ratio of manias to depressions tends to be fairly constant throughout the illness course. If your patient has shown a particular pattern of illness then they will usually continue along the same path. Overall, treatments for mania are probably more effective than those for depression so that in the long term the problem you will be faced with as a doctor treating bipolar patients is the management of chronic depression.

2.22 How often does mania switch into depression?

Up to a third of manias end in depression and a similar proportion of manias are preceded by depression. These are not always severe depressions and some level of low mood can be expected after mania – often an understandable reaction when patients recognise how they have been behaving and the consequences of this. It can be difficult to judge when this low mood tips into depression.

Some patients have a regular pattern of switching in their illness so that, for example, they can expect to experience depression after mania (*Fig. 2.7*). Men are particularly likely to have this pattern of illness.

Because of this pattern of switching it is always advisable to be looking at long-term treatment in whichever pole you are treating. The best way of preventing one pole of the illness is to prevent the other!

2.23 How quickly do episodes of mania and depression come on?

'I can go from zero to supernova in 48 hours' is the classic comment about the onset of mania but sometimes the onset is over several weeks and it is

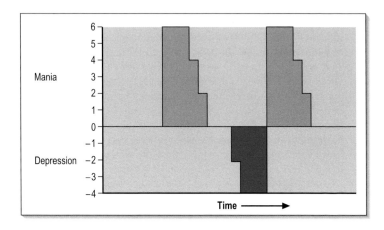

▲

Fig. 2.7 The commonest time for mania and depression to occur is immediately following an episode of the opposite pole.

only as behaviour becomes more extreme that boorish irritable behaviour can be clearly seen to be part of a manic swing. Depression is more commonly insidious in its onset over a few weeks rather than a few days and tends to move from mild to more severe states gradually.

2.24 How many people become chronically depressed?

Depression tends to be the problem that dogs manic depressives in the long term. This is partly because patients recognise depression better than mania as it is a more distressing state to experience (in contrast, families tend to notice more and cope less well with highs). However, it is also true that mild but persistent low mood is the commonest mood state that patients experience, so that on average bipolars can find themselves in a recognisably depressed mood state for a third of the time. Although there is no such term as hypodepression, perhaps there should be as this seems to be one of the commonest and most persistent mood states that bipolars experience. It is this problem which can make a very major difference to the quality of life for manic depressives, and it often goes unnoticed by others because it is not causing an immediate problem or crisis which mania does.

2.25 How can the future course of the illness be predicted?

Past performance is the best predictor of future prospects. It can be very useful to draw up a life chart with a patient (*see Fig. 6.1*) which shows when their illness started, what episodes they have had and what treatment has been taken. Looking at the frequency, severity and type of previous episodes in relation to what medications have been used can indicate a pattern and give some indication of the future. However, if you look very hard it is easy to see patterns that are not really there.

When trying to help someone to predict the future course, look particularly at the well interval for some guidance as to when the next episode is likely to occur. For instance, if someone suffered a period of mania as a student in their twenties and then a period of depression in their forties (*Case vignette 2.2*) it is reasonable to be confident that there will be a further lengthy well interval (*see Q 2.18*). However, strong predictions in manic depression should be avoided as the illness often surprises, both with patients with frequent relapses reaching lengthy stability and others who have been free of the illness for many years experiencing multiple episodes.

The other major factor in prediction is insight – how well has the illness been recognised and what action has been taken to avoid relapse or extra treatment undertaken at an early stage?

CASE VIGNETTE 2.2 A LENGTHY WELL INTERVAL

Martin developed a severe depression 30 years ago at the age of 19 when he was an apprentice electrician. He had to give up the course and spent 3 months in hospital. The admission was lengthy because he became manic during treatment with amitriptyline and so was then given chlorpromazine and slowly recovered. He got back to work after a year but was finding it very difficult to sustain, probably because of low level depressive symptoms. By the end of the next year he was again suffering from depression and was treated with amitriptyline in combination with lithium. He made a good recovery and returned to work, this time in his father's building firm. After a year he reduced and stopped the amitriptyline and the following year decided to try without the lithium. He remained well and built a successful career, eventually taking over the firm from his father.

At the age of 44 Martin again became depressed. Initially this was just feeling low and losing motivation. He was treated with fluoxetine but the symptoms continued to progress, he was losing weight and was unable to concentrate on work which made him feel very anxious. Lithium was added but his condition continued to deteriorate; he stopped eating and was drinking little. He was treated with a course of 10 electroconvulsive therapy treatments which led to recovery from his depression over 5 weeks. He has continued with lithium over the 5 years since then and has been well; he did however decide to let his own son take over more responsibility for the family business.

2.26 Does bipolar II illness develop into bipolar I?

Generally the pattern of bipolar illness for any particular person tends to be fairly constant, both in its severity in each episode and the frequency of episodes. So you would expect that if only hypomanic episodes have occurred that this will be the pattern for the future. However, just as there is a small number of people each year that 'convert' from recurrent unipolar depression to bipolar illness there is also a small number that convert from bipolar II (recurrent depression and hypomania, *Fig. 2.8*) to bipolar I (recurrent depression and mania). This is particularly likely to occur if they are taking high doses of antidepressants (especially if they are not taking lithium) or if the depressions themselves are becoming more severe and so require higher levels of treatment. Stopping treatment such as lithium suddenly can precipitate mania for the first time and that is why it is important to change from treatments only slowly (*see Q 5.27*).

2.27 How common is chronic illness?

About a quarter of those with manic depression will be experiencing symptoms which are so persistent that they are rarely free of them. Most commonly these are chronic depressive symptoms which are at a relatively mild but still distressing and disabling level. There are other patients who become chronically manic although this is rarer. A similarly small proportion continues a relentless course of switching between mania and

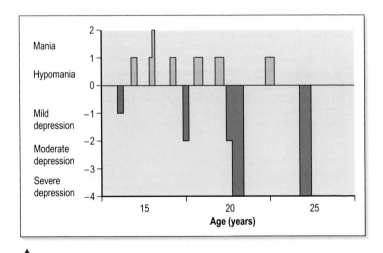

▲

Fig. 2.8 The course of bipolar II illness with hypomania and depression.

depression over days/weeks or months in the longer term (*see Q 1.12*). Although there are not many of these patients about, if you look at any long-term facility for chronically ill psychiatric patients there will be a number of people with manic depression among the larger group with chronic schizophrenia. These patients are commonly women who have started their illness at a rather later age and who also have prominent cognitive impairment.

2.28 Is bipolar disorder a progressive condition?

There is a small increase in the frequency of relapse with time, but this effect is small. It would be expected that each of the first few episodes has a shorter well interval but then usually a more stable pattern emerges (*Fig. 2.9*). However the course of manic depression is endlessly variable!

Those people who have the most severe illnesses will usually suffer frequent relapses and poor recovery right from the start. It is usually apparent from early on who has a better prognosis as they will experience shorter, less severe episodes with a long well interval. However the social

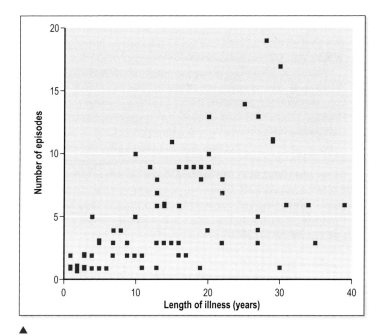

▲
Fig. 2.9 The relationship of the number of episodes to the length of illness.

toll of the illness can grow with time even if the frequency and severity of the episodes do not. Losing close relationships (including divorce, which is particularly likely for manic depressives) and a lack of consistency at work often lead to cumulative personal damage.

2.29 Is manic depression a permanent condition?

The vulnerability to episodes of mania and depression probably lasts a lifetime and having experienced one or more manias and depressions then there is a lifelong vulnerability to recurrence.

There is a small group of between 10 and 20% of people who have suffered several episodes of illness who then have a prolonged period of many years free of bipolar disorder (*see Fig. 2.6*). However it is not uncommon to see people who have been well for many years (*see Case vignette 2.2*) who experience a recurrence 20 years after their last episode. It would appear that the vulnerability to manic depression never goes completely away even when people have been well for many years.

2.30 What is the long term outcome for bipolar disorders?

Professor Angst of Zurich has contributed an enormous amount of information about bipolar disorders and their long term course and outcome. His studies have indicated that at 20 years after the start of their illness, more than two-thirds of manic depressives will still be experiencing disabling problems from their illness (*Table 2.1*) (Angst & Sellaro 2000).

There is no doubt that manic depression is one of the most serious and disabling illnesses to which mankind is subject. The World Health Organization ranks it in the top ten conditions that lead to death and disability. This would seem unlikely at first sight because it is a relatively uncommon illness. However, as it afflicts people from an early age, it has a major impact on working lives and so a considerable economic impact.

2.31 Does bipolar illness develop into dementia/schizophrenia?

There is no evidence that manic depression leads on to dementia. It is true that sometimes the early stages of dementia present with prominent mood symptoms – usually depression but sometimes also of elation. Agitation and restlessness are themselves common symptoms in dementia and can be the presenting complaints early in the illness. There is some evidence of cognitive impairment in manic depression. If this does progress it is a very slow progression and certainly not the rapid progression usually seen in dementia (*see Q 6.3*).

There is a small number of patients who are clearly diagnosed as having manic depressive illness who then develop symptoms that are typical of schizophrenia. After a few years it then becomes clear that they are suffering from chronic schizophrenia rather than manic depression. Some people say

TABLE 2.1 Long term outcome in bipolar disorder		
Outcome	Description	Percentage
Recovered	Good function, no episode in 5 years	16
Remitted	Good function but more than one episode in 5 years	25
Incomplete remission	Impaired function, still recurrent	35
Chronic	More than 2 years in episode	16
Suicide		8

Adapted from Angst & Sellaro (2000).

the diagnosis was wrong to start with and that the manic illness was an early stage of schizophrenia, and if you had searched more carefully you would have found features of schizophrenia. It is very common for those with schizophrenia to suffer prominent symptoms of depression and up to a third experience excited and elated periods but the symptoms typical of schizophrenia continue throughout.

The border between manic depression and schizophrenia is a blurred one, and you will find some psychiatrists who seem to diagnose almost everybody with a psychotic illness as having a schizoaffective disorder as they can find elements of schizophrenia and also of affective illness in every severe mental illness. This doesn't seem to be a very helpful way of proceeding as most trials of treatment are based on one diagnosis or the other and treatment trials in schizoaffective disorder are few and far between. The point of diagnosis is to guide treatment and estimate prognosis and that is why it is worth making the split between the diagnoses. Having said that, there are patients who clearly do stand on the border and merit the diagnosis of schizoaffective disorder (*see Q 1.15*).

2.32 What is likely to trigger off a recurrence?

Most episodes of mania and depression come out of the blue without any clear precipitant.

When you look carefully at stressful life events there is an excess before both depression and mania (*see Fig. 2.4*). However, adverse life events are probably only responsible for about 20% of episodes of mania or depression. There is some evidence that early episodes of an illness are more likely to be triggered by adverse events. It is difficult to tease out the effects of life events from the natural course of the illness. Unpleasant and distressing events happen to all of us (on average three serious events a year) and if you become ill (in any way but particularly psychiatric illness) you will tend to try to find a link to something that has happened recently, in a search for meaning.

It is usually adversity that triggers affective illness although rarely you come across a patient whose illness started after a great success or a very positive event in their life.

> Other well-known precipitants include stopping treatment, in particular suddenly stopping lithium (*see Q 5.27*). Having a baby is a potent precipitant, particularly of mania but also of depression (*see Q 6.17*). Some people also report a seasonal element to relapses of their manic depression (*see Q 2.34*).

2.33 Does the menstrual cycle affect bipolar illness?

Most women who are depressed will notice that their depressive symptoms are worst in the premenstrual phase; this is true in both unipolar and bipolar illness. Likewise some women report improvements in their affective illness when they take the oral contraceptive, although others find that it makes their symptoms worse. Without any good clinical trial data available it is difficult to give any general advice but each case needs to be judged individually. My approach is to focus first on the usual treatments for manic depression and only to consider hormonal approaches if the standard treatments are not effective.

In mania there are no known effects of the menstrual cycle.

It is uncommon for bipolar illness to be diagnosed before menarche in girls or before puberty in boys, suggesting that there is some alteration, which may relate to the hormonal changes occurring at this time that increases the vulnerability to affective disorders.

The potency of childbirth to precipitate both mania and depression is well known (*see Q 6.17*) and this is a common time for the illness to appear. It has been reported that manic depression can arise for the first time at the menopause, but this is rare. There is no clear connection between the illness and the menopause which would allow you to predict for a woman what is likely to occur to her manic depression at this time. Some find that their illness actually improves and they achieve more stability; others report it to be a stormy time for their illness. It can be tempting to try using hormone replacement therapy to alleviate affective symptoms but it is better to focus on the usual treatments at least initially and only experiment with hormonal treatment if this is not successful.

2.34 Does manic depression occur more often at a particular time of year?

There is a condition called seasonal affective disorder where people experience depression starting in the autumn or winter with a recovery by the spring, often accompanied by a hypomanic episode.

However, among those with bipolar I disorder (i.e. depression with mania rather than hypomania) a predictable seasonal relapse is uncommon. In fact even those with seasonal affective disorder often develop depressions or hypomanias at the wrong time of year.

Bright artificial light is an effective treatment for recurrent winter depression (*see* Q 3.34). This approach does require a considerable time commitment: at least an hour in the morning sitting very close to and looking repeatedly at a light. Some people are able to stick with this but most find it difficult to sustain. There are now some 'light hats' – baseball-type caps with lights in the visor – which are easier to use, but look slightly ridiculous and patients should probably be discouraged from going out in them unless they are trying to gain a reputation for eccentricity. Alternatives to the light treatment are walking outside or antidepressant drugs.

2.35 How important is a regular sleep pattern?

Sleep loss is a potent precipitant of mania and so shift work is not a good option for people with manic depression. Maintaining a regular sleep pattern is an important part of manic depressives taking good care of themselves in order to minimise the chance of relapse.

It has been reported that air travel can precipitate mania and most doctors who cover airports will have seen more than their share of manic patients arriving. It has been suggested that those travelling from west to east are more likely to become manic but it is difficult to understand why this should be so. The sleep loss and jet lag are probably both relevant factors in this as the body clocks of bipolars are sensitive to these changes. This needs to be considered by the jet-setting bipolar patient and judicious use of hypnotics to help the adjustment is a good idea.

Most of those who are depressed will be having difficulty sleeping at night but will often resort to sleeping in the day. This can lead to the sleep pattern becoming very erratic. It is worth encouraging the depressed to try to get as much of their sleep as possible at night and not sleep in the day (*see* Q. 3.30).

A proportion of bipolars who are depressed are sleeping excessively and this pattern also exacerbates depression. Again it is very difficult to change this but encouraging them to get up at a reasonable time and not going to bed too early is worthwhile. A more extreme approach of sleep deprivation can be an effective antidepressant treatment both in unipolar and bipolar depression. This involves keeping patients awake all night, usually for 3 or 4 nights (and days). It can lead to a beneficial change in mood but is usually only a short-term solution. Sometimes it is helpful for those with an intractable depression when a shift out of their depression even for a short period can give you and them hope that a change can be made.

 PATIENT QUESTIONS

2.36 What are the chances of my children suffering from manic depression if I do?

The lifetime risk in the general population of developing manic depression is between 1 and 2 in 100. That means that everyone has a 1–2% chance of developing the illness. If you suffer from manic depression then each of your children has about a 10–15% chance of developing this illness. However there is another 15% chance that they will suffer from depression, but not mania. So if you have 10 children probably one will suffer from manic depression, but another one or two will suffer from a serious depression.

Would this be sufficient to deter you from having children? Most people faced with this decision still decide to go ahead and have children, providing they are managing well in their own lives and are in a stable relationship. You have to think about how much the illness has affected you (and so how much it would be likely to affect the life of any child who developed the illness) but also to balance this with what you have achieved in your life.

If both you and your partner have the illness then your children have about a 60–70% chance of having some form of the illness, either depression or mania; again recurrent depression is more common than manic depression.

2.37 What are the chances of getting ill again if I have had only one bout of mania?

The recurrence rate in bipolar illness is very high. If you have had an episode of mania then it is almost inevitable (greater than 90% chance) that you will have a further episode or a depression at some time, though the well interval can be many years. Following a first manic episode the chances of another episode of mania or a depression is about 50:50 in the following year. If you have already had an episode of depression before the mania or have not made a full recovery then the chances are higher. Otherwise it is very difficult to predict whether any particular person at their first illness is more or less liable to recurrence than average.

2.38 If I suffer from hypomania is it likely to develop into more serious mania?

Generally the pattern of bipolar illness for any particular person tends to be fairly constant both in its severity in each episode and the frequency of episodes. So you would expect that if you have only suffered from hypomania then this will be the pattern for the future.

However, some people do change. Those who experience recurrent bouts of depression have about a 10% chance of becoming bipolar, i.e. experiencing their first episode of mania. If you have already had hypomanic episodes then there is a small chance (probably also about 10%) of moving up to mania. It is for this reason that you need to be cautious of taking antidepressants, particularly at a high doses, as these can increase the chance of mania developing. Suddenly stopping lithium is also thought to be a strong precipitant of mania and so if you need to stop lithium you should only do so very gradually over a few weeks.

2.39 Is it likely that I will get further manias or just depressions?

Women are more likely to have an illness that has a preponderance of depression and men more likely to have recurrent manias. However, most patients have a combination of the two. The past pattern of illness including which pole is dominant tends to be consistent for any patient over many years.

2.40 Will the illness get worse as I get older?

There is a small increase in the frequency of relapse with time, but this effect is small. Those people who have the most severe illnesses will suffer frequent relapses and poor recovery right from the start. Those at the milder end of the spectrum will experience shorter, less severe episodes with a long well interval throughout their lives. However, the cumulative effect of the illness can grow with time as each illness compounds the problems that have built up even if the frequency and severity of the episodes are not changing. Relationships breaking up and a lack of consistency at work tend to be the most common causes of the cumulative personal damage.

2.41 Will it ever go away?

Once you have developed manic depression the propensity to the illness probably lasts a lifetime. If you have had one episode you are vulnerable for the rest of your life. If you have had several episodes of the illness at one time in your life it is very likely that you will get them again later in your life.

There is a small group of between 10 and 20% of people who have suffered from manic depression who seem to make a full recovery and have no episodes over many years. Whether the illness has completely gone away is not entirely clear as you also see people who have been well for many years (see Case vignette 2.2) who experience a recurrence 20 years after their last episode. It seems likely that the vulnerability to manic depression never goes away completely even when people have been well for many years.

2.42 Should I avoid stress?

It can be very stressful trying to avoid stress! Making changes to your lifestyle so that you are not putting yourself under excessive pressure at work or in other commitments seems sensible advice. However, it does not make sense to go to the other extreme, pulling out of all commitments and then starting to worry that something might come along that would disrupt the calm. No man is an island and the benefits that come from close personal relationships are usually our most valued. On the other hand, they are also the most likely source of stress and difficulty.

The aim of any plan of treatment is to help people to live as normal a life as they can and do the things they want to do in life. I would not advocate major restrictions unless it is clear from the pattern of the illness that there is no alternative.

Treatment of bipolar depression

3

3.1 What is the best medication for depression in someone who has a history of mania (bipolar I depression)?

 Giving antidepressants on their own to a patient with a history of mania is not to be recommended because antidepressants can precipitate mania (*see Q 3.15*).

Another reason to avoid monotherapy with antidepressants is that the commonest time to become manic is following an episode of depression and consideration should be given to how to prevent this happening. Although antidepressants are the mainstay of treatment for bipolar depression they should only be used in combination with a medication that will prevent mania (*see Q 3.6*).

The first line of treatment for bipolar depression is to consider increasing lithium or other longer term treatment, such as valproate or carbamazepine if this is possible.

3.2 Which antidepressants are the most useful?

The choice of antidepressant should be made in the light of previous treatment and response. Choose an antidepressant that has been helpful and safe in the past over one that has not previously been tried. Unfortunately there have been relatively few trials specifically for bipolar depression so a lot of practice is guided by studies of unipolar depression.

3.3 Which types of antidepressant are commonly available?

Selective serotonin reuptake inhibitors (SSRIs) are the most commonly used antidepressants in the UK. They are not only the first line treatment for unipolar depression but also the first line treatment for bipolar depression. Tricyclic antidepressants are also effective in the treatment of both unipolar and bipolar depression (*Table 3.1*).

The benefits of SSRIs over tryclics are that they are simple to take (usually once daily dosage) and the initial dose is usually an effective dose. In addition, SSRIs are less likely to cause manic switch than tricyclics (*Table 3.2*). In contrast the tricyclics require a gradual increase to an effective dose because of side-effects, usually over at least 2 weeks. The level of side-effects of SSRIs is low and they are relatively safe if taken in overdose.

There have been reports that agitation and suicidal impulses may be increased in the first few weeks on SSRIs (Medicines and Healthcare Products Regulatory Agency 2003). It is difficult to disentangle this effect from a deteriorating depression which is not responding to treatment, as suicidal thoughts are an integral part of depression (*see Q 1.8*).

Response to antidepressants is idiosyncratic and only a proportion (at best two out of three) of patients will tolerate and recover with treatment with SSRIs. The next line of treatment is usually a tricyclic antidepressant.

TABLE 3.1 Antidepressant treatment of bipolar depression

Antidepressant group	Commonly used drugs	Common side effects	Special precautions	Comments
SSRIs	Fluoxetine Paroxetine Sertraline Citalopram	Nausea, agitation, sexual problems	May cause agitation early in treatment	Usual first line treatment
Tryclic antidepressants	Amitriptyline Clomipramine Imipramine	Dry mouth, constipation, drowsiness, weight gain	More likely to precipitate mania	Usual treatment in resistant cases
SNRIs	Venlafaxine Mirtazepine	As with tricyclics, venlafaxine can reduce sleep, mirtazepine is sedative	Raised blood pressure at higher doses of venlafaxine	Mirtazepine has a lower level of sexual side-effects
Dopamine reuptake inhibitor	Buproprion	Dry mouth, insomnia, rarely seizures	Not a licensed anti-depressant in UK	Usual dose 300–400 mg daily Low level of sexual side-effects Useful for smokers?
MAOIs	Moclobemide Phenelzine	Sleep disturbance, headache	Drug interactions and dietary precautions are needed	Older MAOIs need to be used with caution

MAOIs, monoamine oxidase inhibitors; SNRIs, serotonin and norepinephrine reuptake inhibitors; SSRIs, selective serotonin reuptake inhibitors.

3.4 Are there any other types of antidepressant used in the treatment of bipolar depression?

There are other types of antidepressant, two of which are relatively little used in unipolar depression but have been studied in bipolar depression.

MOCLOBEMIDE

Moclobemide (Manerix) has been shown to be effective and to have a low propensity for 'switch' into mania compared to the tricyclic antidepressant

TABLE 3.2 Metanalysis of rate of manic switch

	SSRI	TCA	Placebo
Unipolar disorder	74/10 246 (0.72%)	14/2716 (0.52%)	8/3788 (0.21%)
Bipolar disorder	9/242 (3.7%)	14/125 (11.2%)	2/48 (4.2%)

SSRI, selective serotonin reuptake inhibitor; TCA, tricyclic antidepressant.
From Peet 1994, with permission.

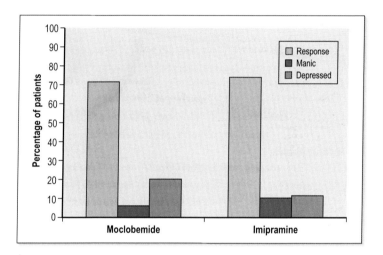

▲

Fig. 3.1 Moclobemide versus imipramine in bipolar depression. (Based on data from Silverstone 2001.)

imipramine (Silverstone 2001) (*Fig. 3.1*). Moclobemide is a monoamine oxidase inhibitor (MAOI) which often worries prescribers because of concerns about dangerous interactions with foods (the cheese reaction occurs when the amino acid tyramine passes through the gut without being broken down and leads to a rise in blood pressure). However, moclobemide is a specific inhibitor of monoamine oxidase in the brain and does not inhibit the form found in the gut. Tyramine can therefore still be broken down in the gut and so does not get through to cause a hypertensive reaction. Moclobemide is also a reversible inhibitor and is relatively short lived so there is only a short (days) wash-out period before another antidepressant can be started if there is a need to change treatment.

BUPROPION

The other unusual treatment is bupropion (amfebutamone) which is not licensed in the UK for the treatment of depression. It is licensed in the UK (as Zyban) as a treatment to increase the success rate in giving up smoking. However, it is commonly used in the United States as an antidepressant at a dose of 300–400 mg daily for unipolar and bipolar depression. It is regarded as an effective treatment for bipolar depression (although trials to date have only been small scale) with a low risk of 'switching' the depression into mania. It may be worth considering if other antidepressants have not been successful or have been poorly tolerated but is usually only prescribed by specialists.

VENLAFAXINE AND MIRTAZEPINE

These drugs are similar in their pharmacological action to the tricyclic antidepressants clomipramine and amitriptyline. All of these drugs work on both serotonin and noradrenaline (norepinephrine) systems in the brain and they are considered to be the most effective antidepressants in unipolar illness if they are taken at a high enough dose. They should certainly be considered in bipolar depression if there is a poor response to other antidepressants.

LAMOTRIGINE

 Lamotrigine, which is only licensed for the treatment of epilepsy, has been shown to be an effective treatment for bipolar depression. However it is not an easy drug to use. The main problem is that it can cause a rash (in about 10%) which occasionally progresses to Stevens–Johnson syndrome. This can require hospital care and is on rare occasions fatal. To reduce the chance of this allergic reaction occurring lamotrigine needs to be introduced very gradually.

Start at 25 mg daily for 2 weeks and then increase to 50 mg daily for the next 2 weeks. The dose can then be increased by 50 mg every 2 weeks, aiming for 200–300 mg daily according to side-effects and response. Because of the slow titration, it can take 3 months to reach an adequate dose and so this is unlikely to lead to a rapid response. However, it does also help to prevent recurrence of bipolar depression without increasing the risk of mania and so can be a very helpful longer term treatment. The usual reason that lamotrigine is prescribed is in manic depression that is dominated by depression which is difficult to treat. Lamotrigine can be introduced as a long-term measure to reduce the frequency and severity of depression and can lead to a considerable long-term improvement.

3.5 For how long should antidepressants be continued after recovery from depression?

The concern for bipolars who continue antidepressants is that they may be running an increased risk of mania while they are on this treatment.

Because of this it would be recommended to discontinue antidepressants at an early stage after recovery from bipolar depression at about 3 months. This is in contrast to the advice for those with unipolar depression which is to continue the antidepressants for at least 6 months after recovery. Unipolar depressives are also often advised to take antidepressants long term as preventive treatment; however this would not usually be appropriate for bipolars.

For bipolars consideration needs to be given to effective long-term preventive treatment such as lithium (*see Chapter 4*). If they are to continue with antidepressants they must also take an antimanic drug, such as lithium, an antipsychotic or valproate (*see Q 3.7*).

It is always worth checking the individual's history – what has been the experience following previous episodes of depression? If this indicates that switching to mania occurred following each depression then the antidepressant should be stopped within a few weeks of recovery from depression.

3.6 Should bipolars continue on their long-term preventive treatment if they become depressed?

Definitely. It is very important that long-term prophylactic treatment (e.g. with lithium) is continued when the patient becomes depressed. This is because the depression is most likely being treated with antidepressants and if the lithium is stopped there is an increased chance of switching into mania (*Fig. 3.2*). Obviously at some point the patient will need to be reviewed to assess how effective the preventive treatment is, but the usual time to do this is after recovery from the acute episode of depression.

3.7 Is there a role for long-term antidepressants as a way of preventing depression recurring in bipolars?

Taking an antidepressant on its own as a preventive treatment in bipolar I disorder is definitely not recommended. However, if an antidepressant has proved beneficial in combination with a mood stabiliser and the previous history has been of a preponderance of depression, then continuing antidepressants is likely to be a good strategy. It may also be worth considering other combinations or alternative mood stabilisers in this situation.

Many bipolar II patients are treated successfully in the long term with antidepressants without lithium or other preventive treatments. This

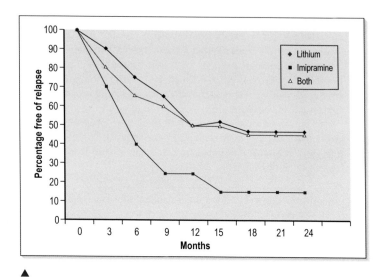

▲

Fig. 3.2 Treatment with lithium in combination with antidepressants reduces antidepressant-induced manic relapse. (From Prien et al 1984, with permission.)

usually follows on from a period of treatment with antidepressants that has been successful without a switch into hypomania. As long as an eye is kept on making sure that elated periods are not occurring, then this is a reasonable option. However, there is a need to be wary as many of those who suffer from hypomanias are not good at recognising them or tend to play down the problems that they cause. Ask someone else in the family if the patient is getting on reasonably.

3.8 What is the best medication for depression in someone who has a history of hypomania but has never been manic (bipolar II depression)?

The mainstay of treatment for bipolar II depression is antidepressants, one option being the SSRI fluoxetine (*Fig. 3.3*). However, the initial decision to be made is whether to prescribe a drug that will prevent manic symptoms developing in addition to the antidepressant. This is a matter of judgement – at one end of the scale a patient who has had only short-lived and not disabling hypomania in the past is suitable for antidepressant treatment on its own but with monitoring for the appearance of manic symptoms. At the other end, someone who is currently depressed but with previous prominent, frequent and socially disabling hypomania should certainly be

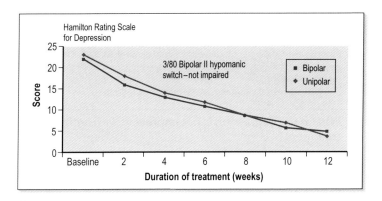

Fig. 3.3 Treatment of depression with fluoxetine in bipolar and unipolar patients. (From Amsterdam et al 1998, with permission.)

taking treatment to prevent further manic symptoms along with the antidepressant. Judging where a patient is on this spectrum is difficult and prescribing treatment often requires a lot of negotiation as many patients will be keen to relieve the depression but may not be concerned about hypomanic symptoms. It is usually the case that the manic depressive patient is very keen to relieve and prevent depression but the family (and others including doctors) are more concerned about the social disruption of hypomania.

The choice of antidepressant for bipolar II depression is the same as that for bipolar I depression (*Case vignette 3.1*).

You need to be wary that treatment with an antidepressant on its own in bipolar II patients may be leading to more instability of mood or even rapid cycling.

CASE VIGNETTE 3.1 ANTIDEPRESSANTS MAY DESTABILISE THE COURSE OF BIPOLAR ILLNESS

Melanie has had periods of depression that began in her twenties. At first they were noticeable because she felt very down and couldn't sleep well but she put these down to the stressful job she was doing which involved a lot of travelling round the country. She had spells like this once or twice a year and they lasted about 6 weeks, and she would often miss a few days' work when she couldn't get out of bed. However, she would always bounce back and often after a bad spell she would feel much better and treat herself a bit, particularly buying designer clothes for which she had a penchant.

A bad spell of depression then hit her and she was off work for a month and started treatment with an antidepressant. This seemed to get her right within a couple of weeks but she went a bit more over the top and to her embarrassment ended up sleeping with one of her salesman who was 10 years her junior. This led to another spell of depression but an increase in the antidepressant again led to improvement. However, by the end of the year she was feeling 'all over the place', never knowing how her mood was going to be week to week. Her work was going badly as she was now regarded as a liability when previously reliability was her middle name.

A trial of lithium without an antidepressant is indicated.

3.9   What if the depression is not improving with antidepressant treatment?

The following questions should be considered before contemplating a change in medication:

- ■ *Have you given the treatment long enough?*: At least 4 weeks with no response, or 6 weeks with only minor response. It can be difficult to stick with the treatment when there is little improvement; a realistic time scale for improvement should be discussed with the patient from the beginning – it may well take up to 4 weeks to start to see a difference. It is also worth discussing at this point the balance between the time needed to give this treatment a good try against the time it will take to make a changeover to another medicine. Focusing on other ways that the patient can help to make a difference to the level of depression is also useful (*see Qs 3.29 and 3.36*).
- ■ *Have you tried a high dose?*: If the patient is not improving, doses should be increased to the maximum, provided that the treatment is reasonably tolerated before turning to an alternative antidepressant.
- ■ *Have you assessed concordance/compliance?*: Is the patient really in agreement with this treatment and taking it (*see also Q 5.43*)? Are they forgetting because they are feeling so tired, lethargic and can't remember to do anything including taking the tablets? Is there some way of improving this – linking it with some more routine or habitual aspect of their life (e.g. brushing their teeth)?
- ■ *Are they physically ill?* (*see Q 3.27*): Specifically, are they hypothyroid or anaemic?
- ■ *Are they drinking alcohol to excess or taking illicit drugs?*
- ■ *Is there another medication that they are taking that might be affecting their depression (e.g. steroids)?*
- ■ *Is there a social or relationship problem that could be addressed?*

3.10   What are the next lines of treatment in bipolar depression that has not responded to the first antidepressant treatment?

If the patient is taking lithium in combination with the antidepressant, first increase the dose of lithium up to a level of about 1.0 mmol/l.

If this is not successful, continue the lithium but change the antidepressant to a different class of drug. It would be worth reviewing what treatments the patient has been on previously to see if it is possible to identify another drug that has been helpful in the past. If no clear treatment option is apparent the usual rule of thumb is that if the patient has been on an SSRI, change to a tricyclic and vice versa.

If the patient is not on lithium then this can be added as an augmenting agent as lithium in combination with antidepressants can lead to more improvement than the antidepressant on its own. (If these options are not successful, this is the stage where most experts are starting to scratch their heads too!)

Other options that are available include other groups of antidepressants, thyroid hormone (at above replacement levels), lamotrigine, tryptophan or electroconvulsive therapy (ECT) (*see Q 3.22*) (*Fig. 3.4*) and psychotherapeutic talking treatments (*see Qs 3.20 and 5.46*).

3.11 Is lithium an effective antidepressant?

Lithium can be an effective treatment for bipolar depression either on its own or in combination with an antidepressant. The first step in treating depression in a manic depressive who is currently on lithium is to check compliance, then the serum lithium level. If there is room to increase the dose of lithium, bearing in mind the blood level and the side-effects, then this should be tried initially unless the illness severity is very high and immediate antidepressant treatment is needed. If the patient is not on lithium, then again this can be a sensible first line treatment as it is likely to be required to prevent a manic swing if the patient is going to be taking an antidepressant.

3.12 Is the treatment for depression in the elderly different?

The same lines of medical treatment are useful for the elderly as for other adults. There is a paradox for the elderly that they are more sensitive to medications in terms of side-effects (probably because of reduced metabolism of drugs, and reduced excretion of lithium) but they also seem to be less responsive to medications and may actually require higher doses.

Physical illness is more likely to complicate treatment in older people which may limit the dose of medicines – for example cardiac disease may limit the dose, or even the prescription of tricyclic antidepressants. ECT is more commonly required in the elderly as they are more likely to experience psychotic symptoms, retardation and poor food and fluid intake.

3.13 Is the treatment for depression in adolescents different?

There are very few trials of treatment of bipolar depression but there are virtually no data on the treatment of bipolar depression in adolescents.

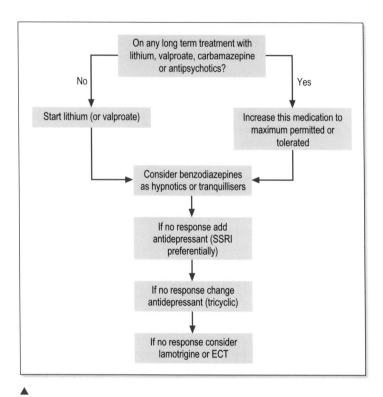

Fig. 3.4 Acute treatment of bipolar depression.

There have been concerns that unipolar depression in this age group does not show a good response to antidepressant medication. This is difficult to reconcile with the data for adults which show a clear benefit in improving depression – is there some basic change in depression and its response to treatment at 18 (or 17)? There are also concerns that some antidepressants (SSRIs) can cause agitation and an increase in suicidal thoughts and behaviour, and that this effect is more marked in adolescents.

Psychological treatment is often recommended for non-bipolar depression in this age group, but unfortunately it is often not available. In bipolar depression there is little evidence to recommend psychotherapeutic approaches on their own.

Overall, even more care needs to be taken when considering the treatment for bipolar depression in adolescents. However, the same lines of treatment as for adults should be followed. Keeping a long-term perspective and focusing on appropriate longer term preventive treatment is a good basic principle, though severe depressive episodes will require antidepressant treatment despite the current uncertainties.

3.14 Should low level depressive symptoms be treated?

As indicated in Chapter 2, chronic depressive symptoms are the most frequent long-term problem for bipolars (*Fig. 3.5*) and we are probably too reticent about treating these. This is partly because it is the manic symptoms that tend to be much more obvious to health professionals and family. Patients may be suffering with low level depressive symptoms but the fact that they are not actually getting into the trouble that occurs in mania can lead one to think that this situation is all right. There is also concern about using antidepressants because of the risk of making the illness worse (*see Qs 3.15 and 6.23*). However, long-term but low-level depressive symptoms do need to be searched for and considered.

■ The first line of treatment is to optimise current medication. If the patient is on long-term treatment such as lithium, there may be leeway to increase this further, provided that side-effects are tolerable and blood levels are not excessive.

■ If the patient is not on an antidepressant and long-term preventive treatment has been maximised, then look at the effects of previous antidepressants. If they have led to a worsening of the illness through rapid cycling or quick switches into mania then antidepressants should only be used with great caution or not at all. Some antidepressants have a lower propensity for inducing mania and so one of these may be more appropriate (*see Table 3.2*).

■ If the patient is taking an antidepressant ensure that this is at a therapeutic dose – just because the symptoms are of a lowish level doesn't mean the antidepressant should also be at a lowish level. It is worth trying to reach the highest dose tolerated with one antidepressant before considering changing to another.

■ Combinations of longer term preventive treatments (e.g. lithium with carbamazepine or valproate) should also be considered.

■ Finally, consider an alternative such as lamotrigine (*see Q 3.4*) which is less likely to lead to the complications of switching and rapid cycling.

3.15 Do antidepressants trigger mania?

Antidepressants can trigger a manic illness in those who have previously been manic, but only rarely in those who have not previously been manic (*see Table 3.2*). Antidepressants should not be prescribed to someone who has had a previous episode of mania (even if it was a long time ago) without an additional treatment to prevent mania.

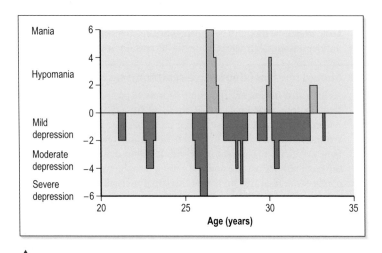

▲

Fig. 3.5 Bipolar disorder dominated by depression.

Tricyclic antidepressants are more likely to trigger mania than SSRIs. The use of antidepressants of all types is also associated with rapid cycling (several episodes of mania and depression in quick succession). Patients who have a rapid cycling pattern should not continue to take antidepressants and stopping these drugs can lead to a considerable improvement in the stability of their mood.

Whether it is reasonable to give antidepressants to someone who has only suffered hypomania but not mania in the past is much more uncertain. It is not clear whether antidepressants can lead to mania in someone who has only been hypomanic previously. One trial in this group of patients found that some did become hypomanic again, but did not find that patients became manic for the first time (Amsterdam et al 1998) (*see Fig. 3.3*)

The safest line of treatment would be the combination of an antidepressant with lithium but patients who have experienced hypomanias but not manias are often reluctant to take antimanic medications.

3.16 What treatment is needed for depression with psychotic symptoms?

It is usually only the most severe depressions that are accompanied by psychotic symptoms. Psychotic depression is a high risk state and the propensity to suicide is very high in this group, and they are more unpredictable. They often need treatment in hospital and a high degree of nursing care, not just for their safety but also because they have difficulty looking after their basic needs, including feeding and washing.

These more extreme depressive states will frequently warrant treatment with ECT (*see Q 3.22*).

> Psychotic depression requires treatment with both antidepressants and antipsychotics. There is also a substantial risk of shifting into mania from the psychotic depressed state and so the antipsychotic drug needs to be continued at least as long as the antidepressant.

3.17 What is the best treatment for anxiety symptoms in bipolar depression?

Anxiety symptoms occur commonly and often prominently in bipolar depression. They may appear on their own but are more usually part of the depression. The first line of treatment would be to treat the anxiety symptoms as if they are an aspect of depression (*see Q 1.14*). However, the anxiety symptoms may persist despite antidepressant treatment at a full dose in combination with a mood stabiliser. If there are still prominent depressive symptoms then follow the usual further lines for treating depression (*see Qs 3.10 and 6.21*). It is worth giving some consideration to the antidepressant being prescribed as MAOIs are thought to be more effective in depression with anxiety.

Pragmatically, many doctors treat prominent anxiety symptoms with antipsychotics and these certainly can produce a calming effect for many patients. The dilemma when doing this is leaving the patient relatively free of anxiety but sedated because of the antipsychotics, particularly when using the older antipsychotics such as chlorpromazine. The risk of tardive dyskinesia in the long-term use of antipsychotics should also be borne in mind.

Benzodiazepines are commonly prescribed for bipolar patients with prominent anxiety but their use must always be balanced with the likelihood of tolerance and dependence developing. They should only be used for intractable anxiety and only for short periods if possible; however they remain an option. Buspirone is a non-benzodiazepine antianxiety medication. There have been no trials of this medication in bipolar patients but it may be worth considering and some patients have responded well to this in combination with an antidepressant.

There are effective psychological techniques and treatments that are beneficial for anxiety symptoms:

■ Has the patient read a book about managing anxiety effectively? (*see Further reading*).

■ Is there a local psychologist or cognitive therapist who could help to teach these techniques? (*see also Q 3.21*).

3.18 How is the risk of suicide judged?

This is a challenge for everyone who looks after manic depressives, and the statistics on suicide – that between 10 and 25% of those suffering from manic depression die through suicide – are very sobering and confirm our limited capacity to judge suicide risk and to prevent it.

It is important to focus on the more immediate basis for judgement of risk by considering what the patient is saying at the time they are seen. However, to get a full picture, several background factors should be taken into account:

■ All those suffering from manic depression are at least at moderate risk for suicide – this serious mental illness substantially inflates the risk. It is not justifiable to regard anyone with this diagnosis as at low risk for suicide.

■ The quality of the patient's life is usually based on having close relationships, employment, financial security and physical health. These aspects of life are adversely affected in those who do commit suicide but are very difficult to change.

■ Older age is a risk factor for suicide in the general population but is less important among manic depressives where suicide occurs across the age range.

■ Personality factors – including impulsiveness (which can be indicated by previous self-harm, drug and alcohol misuse) – and erratic relationships are also worth considering.

The more immediate factors are usually those that are more susceptible to change – for example what is the current level of depression? Both acute and chronic depressives are at high risk and there may be treatment options that could reduce the level of depression and so the risk of suicide. Recent adverse events also increase the likelihood of suicide but with time the impact of even the worst event (e.g. a close bereavement) tends to abate.

Most people who commit suicide do so when they are intoxicated with alcohol – often because they use it for Dutch courage to carry out a frightening act or to dull the pain of it. Others do not intend suicide when they start to drink but then become more impulsive and reckless when they are drunk. Prediction of risk of suicide in the intoxicated is particularly difficult, though it is invariably higher than when sober.

3.19   How can suicidal ideas be elicited?

Discussing suicidal ideas is never easy, but it does get easier the more you do it. Try to normalise the discussion by making it clear you anticipate that people who are depressed do think about dying and suicide:

■ 'Almost everyone who is depressed feels suicidal at times – I was wondering to what extent this has been affecting you?', followed up by:
■ 'What had you thought you might do?' (Try to find out if the patient has actually made any plans or done any preparatory acts, e.g. putting a noose in the boot of the car.)
■ What does the patient think would be the effect of their suicide on others – from 'I know I couldn't, it would kill my mother' to 'They would all be better off without me, even my baby – then someone would take proper care of her'.
■ What has prevented them from taking their own life? Sometimes the reasons will be a surprise: 'I couldn't stand my ex-wife finally getting the house!'

The usual block is either consideration of others or not having the courage to go through with it. Has the patient actually done something already that could have been fatal, or was intended to be fatal? Be wary of dismissing those who have committed multiple previous suicidal-type acts such as frequent overdoses – these people are at higher not lower risk and are more likely to finally kill themselves.

The presence of psychotic ideas or experiences makes successful suicidal acts more likely. Using the usual judgements about their ideas on psychotic depressives is very risky as these are the patients that are most likely to surprise you as it is not possible to use logic on those for whom logic has gone out of the window.

The other side of the balance in judging suicide risk is: Are there good lines of treatment and care that are likely to make a major difference to the patient's mental illness? It is likely that you would take more extreme action (including detention and enforced treatment if absolutely necessary) in a young person early on in their illness history with an acute severe depression who is very likely to respond to treatment than someone with a history of chronic treatment-resistant depression even if the risk of suicide is similar. It can be easy to concentrate on taking action to prevent suicide – having the family watch the person carefully or admission to hospital – instead of focusing on treatments that are likely to beneficial.

It is worth bearing in mind that a majority of manic depressives who do kill themselves are not on optimal treatment, although this is often because of poor compliance. Lithium does reduce the rate of suicide, some have claimed even to the level of the general population. Has this patient had the best treatment available, or at least a trial of treatments (including lithium) that are known to be beneficial?

It is very unusual for people who are manic to commit suicide. They can, however, hurt themselves through the risks that they take or by overestimating their physical prowess – for example thinking they can run as fast as a train and putting this to the test with tragic results.

3.20 Is psychological treatment for depression useful for bipolars?

The symptoms of bipolar depression can be so disabling with retardation and overwhelming negativity that it is difficult for psychological treatment to penetrate these barriers. However, this line of treatment is worth considering, particularly in the longer term. Several psychological approaches can be helpful and it is usually a combination of approaches, tailored to the individual patient, that is the most successful.

■ *Cognitive behaviour therapy*: This is the mainstay of psychological treatment for depression and the principles of this can be applied in bipolar depression in a manner similar to the way it is used in unipolar depression (*see Q 3.21*). The main differences lie in the fact that the symptoms of mania (e.g. optimistic thinking) may be a bad sign rather than a good one.

■ *Past experiences and relationships*: Other psychological approaches focus more on past experiences and relationships. The aim of this is to help patients to understand the patterns of their relationships, what difficulties have emerged and how their attitudes and feelings have contributed to this. A better understanding can lead to an improvement in relationships.

■ *Marital therapy*: For those who are currently in a relationship, particularly one that is under strain, a good approach to psychological treatment is one that involves the partner as well. Couple or marital therapy can be a very effective way of mobilising the resources of the couple to improve their relationship and making use of the major asset that comprises a good relationship.

■ *Counselling*: This is aimed at resolving current practical and emotional problems. Time is given to looking at ways of managing practical problems – for example a young mother looking at what possibilities there might be for childcare to allow some time away from looking after children. However, it is very difficult for those who are more than mildly depressed to make use of this approach because their negative view of themselves and their situation strongly colours their perception of the problems.

- *Education*: The most basic form of psychotherapy is education, both about the illness in general and about the particular pattern of illness in that patient. It is only when people are able to recognise how the illness manifests itself in their case that they can really take on productive approaches to taking care of themselves and finding which treatments are helpful. This is vital for everyone who suffers from manic depression.

The approaches outlined above can all prove useful for those with bipolar depression; however there has been relatively little research into what specific treatments are most effective for those with manic depression. Hopefully this will become clearer in the next few years, but it is likely that the non-specific factors in psychotherapy are equally as important, including an accepting, understanding, empathic relationship with a therapist who can instil a sense of hope and build on the strengths of the person.

3.21 What is cognitive behaviour therapy?

Cognitive behaviour therapy (CBT) aims to help people to recognise and alter the patterns of behaviour and thinking that occur in depression. There are a variety of approaches used to look at the way people who are depressed talk to themselves inside their heads.

RECOGNISING AND MANAGING NEGATIVE THINKING

This is one of the basic techniques of cognitive therapy. It involves identifying those negative thoughts which spring into the mind easily – for example 'I'm useless' is a classic idea that occurs to a depressive in response to any difficulty. This can lead on to ruminations about how others would be 'better off if I wasn't around' and then to suicidal thoughts. This run of thinking inevitably further depresses the mood and half an hour going round this theme will make anyone feel a lot worse.

- *Step 1*: Recognising this pattern is the first step in intervening – even a simple self-acknowledgement of what is happening can help to stop the rumination. These thoughts are likely to emerge again as they become so automatic, but if active rumination can be changed to an attempt to interrupt, this can be very helpful. There are usually a number of similar 'mental grooves' that make up depressive thinking.
- *Step 2*: The next step after recognition is examining the truth of the self-talk. What does 'I'm useless' mean? Does this mean that the person can't do anything at all – not even make someone a cup of tea?

Usually the automatic depressive thinking is very extreme and it is not difficult for a therapist to challenge it in this way, and usually patients feel better when this is done in an interview.

■ *Step 3*: The third step for patients to learn is to challenge their own thinking; psychotherapy techniques aim to get patients to take this on for themselves. Cognitive therapists have a wide variety of techniques to help people manage their thinking more effectively, but it can also be useful for doctors to use this type of approach in discussions with the depressed (*see Further reading*).

PROMOTING PRODUCTIVE BEHAVIOURS

It is common for those who are depressed to restrict their life to minimal activities, which is often just the essentials – 'the grind'. Even when it is difficult to penetrate the negativity of thinking it can be worth trying to encourage patients to look at what they are doing day by day. Looking at getting back into routines, but starting at a low level, is a first step. Even small changes – having a shower each morning, taking a short walk –can help self-esteem and break into the pattern of inactivity.

Consider also pleasurable activities in which patients had previously been involved and which could be tried out again. Starting with low level activities – a walk in the park with a friend rather than a wild night out on the town – is a sensible place to begin (*see also Q 3.36*).

3.22 Does ECT have a place in the treatment of manic depression?

A few patients who have had ECT in the past and found it to be the most effective treatment will come and ask for this treatment first line if they become depressed. This would be completely outside some guidelines (e.g. National Institute for Clinical Excellence, *see Appendix 1*), but it is a request that should be seriously considered as ECT is the quickest and most effective antidepressant treatment.

Usually, however, ECT is reserved for more extreme situations. The commonest of these would be the treatment of psychotic depression which is life-threatening, either because of suicide risk or where the patient is not eating or drinking sufficiently.

Often those patients in such extreme states lack the capacity to consent to treatment with ECT and occasionally they will agree because they see it as a punishment and this fits with their desire to be punished. Therefore this treatment will often need to be done in a legal context which protects both patients and doctors. In England and Wales this would be with the patient detained under the Mental Health Act 1983 and a second-opinion psychiatrist appointed by the Mental Health Act Commission having agreed with this line of treatment.

Occasionally ECT can be used in the treatment of mania or mixed affective states (*see Q 4.12*).

3.23 What is ECT?

Electroconvulsive therapy (ECT) is the quickest and most effective treatment for depression. However, it is often seen as a barbaric treatment, mainly because the idea of having an electric current applied to your brain is a very worrying one. It is certainly true that unmodified (no anaesthetic and no muscle relaxant) ECT did lead to very serious side-effects including broken bones and has been vividly depicted in the movies. Unmodified ECT is no longer given. The reality of ECT for most patients is that they report it to be only mildly unpleasant and are usually very relieved that their depression is improving.

ECT involves stimulating the brain so that an epileptic convulsion is induced. This is done with a high frequency electrical pulse delivered between two electrodes placed on the scalp. In bilateral ECT the electrodes are placed on opposite sides of the head; in unilateral ECT one electrode is on the side of the head and the other on the top of the head. The non-dominant hemisphere (usually the right side) is stimulated in unilateral ECT.

The process of modified ECT involves a general anaesthetic, followed by a paralysing muscle relaxant and then the application of the electric current. Many patients do not realise that they are going to be unconscious and relaxed when they are having the treatment. The treatments are usually given twice a week and a typical course is of between 6 and 12 treatments.

3.24 What are the side-effects of ECT?

 Bilateral ECT is more effective than unilateral ECT but also has more side-effects. The most common side-effect is headache and most patients would experience a mild headache after ECT. The commonest troublesome side-effect is memory loss: this is usually for some of the time around the ECT but can be more extensive. Some patients find this very distressing and all patients should be warned of this possibility. It is difficult to disentangle this side-effect from the effect of depression on memory which is also substantial.

3.25 What are the risks of ECT?

The risks are mainly those of having a general anaesthetic and there are rare deaths associated with ECT, usually when a very debilitated, poorly nourished and dehydrated depressed patient is being treated. This needs to be balanced by the effectiveness of the treatment and the need to provide rapid relief to patients in mental and physical extremis.

3.26 Is transcranial magnetic stimulation a useful treatment for bipolar depression?

Transcranial magnetic stimulation (TMS) involves placing a strong electromagnet next to the skull in order to affect the nerve cells underneath. There have been reports that this can be helpful in treating depression among those with both unipolar and bipolar depression, but the effect is only small and probably temporary. As with many studies of antidepressant effects, the main thrust of research has been on unipolar depression and there is still too little evidence to recommend this treatment in bipolar depression.

Intriguingly, it has been suggested that stimulation over the left prefrontal cortex may improve depression and over the right prefrontal area may alleviate mania. This tallies with other studies of patients who have had a cerebrovascular accident that has led to affective disorder, which also suggests that the illness may lateralise in this way.

The effect of TMS does not appear to be very strong and it seems unlikely that TMS is going to be a commonly used treatment in the near future. In addition, the availability of machines for this purpose is still very limited (Boniface & Ziemann 2003).

3.27 Are there any blood tests or other investigations that should be done when someone is depressed?

Usually bipolar depression comes within a longer course of bipolar disorder. If the patient is taking longer term prophylactic treatment, it is likely that some investigations will have been done, particularly thyroid function tests, as part of monitoring this treatment. However, it is worth bearing in mind that depression can be associated with a variety of physical illnesses. The most important investigation would be a simple review of physical systems to elicit any symptoms indicative of a physical illness. Thyroid function should certainly be checked in any episode of depression. Prominent physical symptoms such as tiredness may prompt investigations to ensure that anaemia is not present. One of the major complications of depression is alcohol misuse and review of liver function may be indicated. It is likely that an estimation of renal function has already been obtained if prophylactic treatment such as lithium is being considered.

3.28 What is the best way to talk to someone who is depressed?

There is no best way but there are aspects of the interview that are worth considering. The depressed often need more time than we usually put aside for consultations, they may be retarded and have poor concentration which means that getting them to provide the relevant information can be slow. They are, however, often easy to deal with briefly because their low self-esteem and hopelessness means that they do not want to take up any time as they don't believe they will be able to get help. The hopelessness of depression can be infectious and there is a need to guard against falling in with this and not following a line of treatment that may be beneficial.

The patient will only be able to take in a small amount of information, so advice needs to be kept simple and should probably be written down as well. It is often helpful to have a friend or relative along as they will be able to recall more from this interview. They can also help to keep a more balanced picture of the meeting than the negative bias that the patient will tend to recall of what has been discussed. Keeping a balance between optimism and realism is difficult, as encouragement should be provided, but unrealistic promises about the benefits of treatment or overoptimistic prognoses for the speed and extent of improvement can backfire later and lead to patients losing confidence in their treatment. Focusing on what someone can do to improve their own symptoms and situation and not just relying on the medication is important (*see Q 3.36*), particularly in helping to improve self-esteem:

- Focusing on the efforts that they have already made and trying to get patients to spell this out can help to get a more realistic view of the current position.
- Looking at what happened during previous periods of depression and how recovery occurred is useful and realistic in terms of prognosis.
- Making plans on an achievable and gradual basis even from a small start – for example having a walk to the post box each day as a beginning on which to build – can discourage unrealistic goals (e.g. walking 5 miles a day, when the post box has not yet been achieved).
- Helping to recognise the circular patterns of thinking and trying to put aside worries even for a short while is helpful.
- Letting patients discuss at length the way they are feeling and the thoughts that they are getting can prove counterproductive and many depressed people complain that counselling makes them feel worse if all they do is talk about their feelings and problems and reinforce their own negativity.

Being listened to is valued by most people who are depressed and it is worth giving some time to this in most interviews – sometimes it can be the major intervention. However, usually there are several assessment and management goals in the interview and there is a need to guard against spending all the time listening and not achieve any of these goals. Getting this balance right is not easy in any consultation, especially when under pressure from time.

Patients will gain confidence if they perceive that their depression is understood – for example by asking about common symptoms that they will have and also understanding that they are likely to be feeling worthless, hopeless and desperate. Accepting that they are likely to have thoughts about death and suicide makes a discussion of these issues much more productive than if they think that you are going to be shocked by these ideas. There are limits to what can be offered but letting patients have a means of contact if they are getting worse – and knowing how quickly they will get a response – can be very helpful.

3.29 What general advice can be given to someone who is depressed?

The suggestions below have a reasonably firm foundation for unipolar depression but there are precious few studies in bipolar depression. However, extrapolation of these ideas to manic depressives with some reservations is worth considering.

DIURNAL RHYTHMS

Most people who are depressed lose the basic rhythm of life, they are sleeping badly and are often up at night whereas in the daytime they are resting, sleeping or doing little. Endocrine studies (e.g. cortisol levels) reflect this as they tend to show that the depressed lose their diurnal rhythm with a constant high level of corticosteroids. Are there small changes that they can make to try to re-entrain themselves so that they are active in the day and thereby give themselves a better chance of sleeping at night?

EXERCISE

Exercise can improve mood – those that exercise regularly have better mental health and trials of exercise in depression have shown the benefit. Those who give up exercise run a higher risk of experiencing depression. No specific trials have been done in bipolar depression but many people report that this is helpful.

To most people exercise implies running or other high exertion sports. Suggesting this to a depressed patient is likely to be ignored when they feel they can hardly get out of bed. Find out what they had been doing before they were depressed or what they used to do earlier in their lives. People are more likely to take up exercise in which they had previously been active rather than try something new. Look initially at low level exercise: doing some walking or going for a swim can be both useful and acceptable. If patients can then build on this to take some exercise regularly at a more substantial level it is likely to be of considerable benefit to their mental and physical health in both the short and the long term.

ENJOYABLE ACTIVITY

Many people who are depressed have brought their range of activities down to the bare minimum – 'just the grind' – and have stopped doing the things that brought pleasure to their lives. Asking 'What do you do for fun?' usually elicits the response that they 'don't do fun' nowadays but can lead on to a discussion of what they had previously done for interest. Again start low and build up rather than have expectations that are unlikely to be achieved.

LIGHT AND SUNLIGHT

Winter depression can be specifically treated with bright light, but many people find the dark winters depressing (*see also* Q 3.34). It is surprising how much light there is outside on even a dull winter's day. Encouraging the depressed to get some fresh air and sunlight, even in the winter, may sound very traditional advice but works for some!

3.30 What advice can be given to someone who is sleeping badly?

It is worthwhile for those suffering from manic depression to have as good a sleep pattern as they can and a variety of techniques to hand that promote sleep. A regular sleeping habit is a good starting point, always going to bed and getting up at the same time. Encouraging people to get up in the morning even if they have not slept well is a good foundation. Sleeping in the daytime tends to make the night's sleep worse but can be very tempting!

Taking some exercise, such as having a walk in the early evening, can improve the chances of getting off to sleep later. Although alcohol can help people get off to sleep it tends to wake them up in the middle of the night as the alcohol levels are coming down. Stimulants such as caffeine in coffee or tea should be avoided in the evening.

There are a variety of techniques that people can use to help to get themselves off to sleep, or at least to relax. Virtually everyone who suffers from manic depression will benefit from having one of these strategies available to them. Relaxation techniques (e.g. breathing exercises) are the most basic methods. These can give both physical and mental relaxation; however it can also be helpful to have a specific mental technique to quieten down the thoughts that are crowding round the mind (*see* Q 3.38). It is generally much easier to learn these techniques when reasonably well rather than when in the grips of depression.

In acute depression with serious sleep problems there are several pharmacological options. If the patient is already on a sedative medication it may be appropriate to increase this – for example raising the dose of carbamazepine at night. If an antipsychotic is being taken the dose of this could be increased or this treatment could be given on a temporary basis – for example olanzapine (usually 5–10 mg) or chlorpromazine (up to 100 mg).

Prescribing a hypnotic is another option, though many are reluctant to use benzodiazepines because for every 10 patients started on them one is likely to continue long term. However, if this is a short-term prescription only then temazepam 10–20 mg is appropriate. The newer sleeping pills such as zopiclone (7.5 mg) are thought to be less likely to lead to dependence but still need to be used with caution.

3.31 How long does an episode of depression usually last?

Even severe episodes of depression do usually remit. If this is the first episode of depression, it is possible to predict with confidence that the patient will recover. Even without treatment the depression will come to a spontaneous end, and prior to modern treatments it was unusual to stay depressed for more than a few months. Looking at how long episodes have lasted previously is a good indicator of how long this one will last.

With the appropriate treatment some improvement should be seen within a month. If there is no improvement on the current treatment after 6 weeks then it is unlikely that this treatment at this dose is going to work. It is, however, worth persevering with each treatment (though not usually each dose) for at least 6 weeks to judge whether the medication is useful. It is very easy to change treatments after a couple of weeks because the symptoms are not improving only to find after three changes that the options are running out and you don't know whether to go back to an earlier treatment!

3.32 When should someone who is depressed be in hospital?

ADVANTAGES

The main advantage of being in hospital is that nursing care is readily available. This gives a good opportunity for assessment of the severity of the depression and its complications including nutrition, hydration and suicide risk. In the most severe cases nursing care includes helping the patient to maintain basic self-care – for example bathing, changing clothes and help with eating and drinking. Nursing staff can also encourage a simple daily routine to try to reinstate a more normal rhythm of activity in the day and sleep at night. Taking away some of the day-to-day responsibilities from those incapable of dealing with them is helpful in the short term.

The usual reason for admission is a combination of how disabled the patient is balanced by the presence of what help is available at home. The lonely isolated depressed man is likely to require admission at a lower severity than the woman with a close family who is able to give the considerable time and sympathetic assistance that is needed by the severely depressed.

DISADVANTAGES

Treatment in hospital can undermine patients who have taken pride in managing despite their depression and can lead to further loss of self-esteem. Life in hospital is rarely calm and peaceful – everyone admitted is in an extreme mental state and being surrounded by disturbed patients can be very disturbing! It can be very hard to get a night's sleep in a ward with even one manic patient who does not want anyone else to be asleep. Some patients can be very disruptive to recovery and encourage others to behave more extremely (e.g. by self-harm such as cutting themselves) or to undermine outside relationships. Remember that being depressed leaves people very vulnerable to others. Illicit drugs are commonly available in and around hospitals; drug dealers often target such patients knowing of their vulnerability.

Coming into hospital and so avoiding dealing with serious problems at home is a double-edged sword. It can be useful to be protected from the difficulties in the real world but it can also lead to those problems escalating – for example as the bills mount up and the electricity is cut off or the flat is vandalised because it is unoccupied. The same is true of relationships that are under strain and a hospital admission can be the final straw that leads to break up.

TO HOSPITALISE OR NOT?

If it is possible to provide extra help at home through the local mental health and social services then this would usually be preferable, unless there is a very high suicide risk or it would put an unreasonable burden on the family. The presence of psychosis in depression is a very ominous sign and it is very likely that admission will be needed unless there is an equivalent level of support outside hospital. There is always a substantial suicide risk among the severely or chronically depressed and judging when this is so high as to require monitoring by nursing staff in hospital is a challenge for us all (*see Q 3.18*). The fact that there is a substantial number of patients who commit suicide during their admission or soon after discharge is testimony to this.

3.33 What advice can be given to relatives of someone who is depressed?

The main advice that can be given to family or friends who are caring for someone with bipolar depression is similar to that given to patients (*see Q 3.36*). It is very helpful to have a family member in the interview when giving advice to a depressed patient because they have such difficulty concentrating and remembering what has been discussed. The discussion will often turn to the balance between trying to encourage the depressed person but not feeling that you are bullying or nagging them. This is a difficult but important balance to strike. Sometimes it is possible to get the patient to tell their carer what they find most helpful and what they want the family to do when they are finding it difficult to motivate themselves. It is more likely to be acceptable when they have initiated the idea rather than when they are being pushed by the relative.

The other worry of carers is suicide risk and this should be discussed as frankly as possible, recognising that suicidal ideas are very common in depression but trying to help carers to identify when this might be becoming too extreme or dangerous for them to manage safely at home (*see* Q 3.19).

Family members need to take care of themselves too – simply asking them how they are getting on can help to acknowledge the major task in which they are involved. Acknowledge the difficulties they face and the range of emotions (including feeling angry) that they are likely to be experiencing – this can help to reduce the guilt they usually feel. Encourage them to find time for themselves away from caring. This can be particularly difficult if they are worried that the depressed person might do something suicidal – help them to look at these risks realistically and to understand that they cannot watch someone every moment.

3.34 What is seasonal affective disorder?

Seasonal affective disorder (SAD) is winter depression often associated with summer hypomania. It is quite a common pattern of bipolar illness, particularly at the milder end of the spectrum. Most of us find some change in our mood and energy between summer and winter – seasonal affective disorder seems to be a magnification of this effect. It may be more common in more northerly climes where the winter night is longer and daylight is in short supply. Like many bipolar depressions it is associated with an increase in appetite and sleep. Some people think it may be related to hibernation in other animals but there is no evidence that any of our animal ancestors hibernated so this is unlikely.

If seasonal affective disorder is related to lack of sunlight then it makes sense to replace this with artificial light (*see also* Q 2.34). There are several types of artificial light boxes available. However, the principle is for the depressed patient to sit next to a very bright light, usually for an hour in the morning and an hour in the evening. They can read a book or be watching television but need to look at the light frequently while they are doing this. This is actually very restrictive and compliance with the treatment is often poor; however some people particularly like this approach. There are now some 'light hats' available which are essentially baseball caps with bulbs in the peak; however, the efficacy of this has not been well proven compared to the light box. The other alternative for getting more light is to have a walk outside as even dull days produce a lot of light and the exercise can also be helpful for depression.

Certainly some patients find light treatment very beneficial and in the UK some will start using it when the clocks go back an hour at the end of British summertime to prevent the onset of their depression. Boxes usually cost about £200 which can be prohibitive for some patients and few clinics hire them out.

3.35 What advice can be given about work when someone is depressed?

This decision is usually easy in bipolar depression as the illness tends to be markedly disabling, with concentration and memory as well as motivation reduced. Often the depression is seriously interfering with even basic functioning such as finding the motivation to get out of bed.

The more difficult decision is when the depression is improving: does one wait for a full recovery or encourage the patient to get back to work early? Feelings of guilt and excessive worry can make this more difficult as the patient wants to get back quickly as they feel they are letting everyone down or they are frightened that they will lose their job. Alternatively, they might be excessively anxious about work and how they will be seen by other people and therefore too reluctant to return.

Try to judge what level of concentration and attention is needed for the job: can this be matched to what they are doing day to day? Is the patient able to read the paper or a book, get jobs done round the house, do any studying? These can be useful pre-work targets. Ascertain if the patient can sustain these over a reasonable period of at least a couple of weeks. Is there a possibility of a gradual return to work, both in terms of time and responsibility?

Many people are concerned that returning to work could make them ill again. If there are specific problems and stresses at work then these need to be dealt with and there are situations where it is clear that returning to work is not an option. However, if there has been a good recovery, try to encourage the patient to return to their previous level of function in every arena. It is usually only getting back to work that gives people the confidence that they can do it, and the work itself helps them to rehabilitate. Do discuss with the patient what to say to colleagues at work; if an answer can be prepared beforehand, this can make life much easier (*see Q 3.41*).

Patients with particularly responsible jobs such as doctors will require assistance from occupational health physicians and often need to move into posts that provide some supervision if they are to work safely.

There is also the need to judge the risk of the patient becoming manic, particularly if this is the previous pattern of illness, and a longer period of mood stability may be required.

PATIENT QUESTIONS

3.36 What can I do to help my depression apart from taking medicines?

Most people who are depressed lose the basic rhythm of life, sleeping badly at night and feeling exhausted in the day and so doing very little. Your internal hormone levels usually vary over 24 hours but this rhythm also gets lost when you are depressed and can make you feel tired and unwell. Are there small changes that you can make to get your daily rhythm back? If you usually go to the shops or visit a friend on a Monday try to keep that going. If you are active in the day you will give yourself a better chance of sleeping at night.

Exercise can improve mood. Exercise can mean anything from walking round the block for 10 minutes to playing in a rugby match. Start small and then try to build up. Find something that you can sustain – it's much better to do a 10-minute walk every day than an hour's run but only as a one off. Walking and swimming are the commonest ways that people start. Getting someone else to come with you is usually very good for motivation. Is there some sport which you used to enjoy? Even if you don't play you could go and watch. Try and get out in the sun and air even if you don't feel that you can go out for a walk.

Many people who are depressed have brought their activities down to the minimum – 'just the grind'. What did you used to do for fun or interest? It is difficult to enjoy yourself if you are depressed but if you never do anything enjoyable then you may not be giving your mood a chance to lift.

3.37 How can I recognise early that the depression is returning?

Most people have a particular depression 'signature'. Each time they become depressed the same symptoms emerge and in a similar pattern. Can you recognise what the pattern is for you? If you find this difficult then look at the common symptoms of depression and try to remember which symptoms came first. It may be that these early symptoms are not particularly important in themselves but they are ones that are apparent in the early days of relapse. For example feeling anxious when you are getting on the bus may be an early sign but something that you are able to deal with effectively. However, if it is a warning sign then it is worth remembering and reacting to.

Ask your family what they have noticed – for example they may have seen that you were starting to get very negative about your job when usually you enjoy it. Encourage them to let you know when they see this happening. You don't have to react immediately to these signs and many people would wait to see if they persist for a week or two before taking any action. You can also end up continually noticing minor symptoms that do not come to anything but worrying unduly about them. There is a balance between recognising early and being overvigilant.

Certain symptoms may be particularly important: sleep loss is usually a serious sign and you should not have more than a couple of sleepless nights before you do something about this. It may be well worth having some medication readily available to deal with sleep problems. Other very ominous signs are symptoms of psychosis (e.g. your ideas become very extreme or you experience hallucinations). These symptoms require treatment as soon as they arise and you should not wait to see what happens.

The other side of recognising the depression returning is having a plan as to what you will do about this, both in terms of medication and your general approach.

3.38   How can I improve my sleep?

You need to have as good a sleep pattern as you can and to have some techniques available that can promote sleep. A regular habit is a good starting point, always going to bed and getting up at the same time. It is very tempting to stay in bed in the morning if you have slept badly the night before, but in the long run you may be making the pattern of your sleep worse. Sleeping in the daytime is the other pattern to try to avoid; if you really can't stop this then try to limit it to a certain length of time, perhaps just an hour. Taking some exercise, such as having a walk in the early evening, can improve the chances of getting off to sleep later. Although alcohol may help you to get off to sleep it tends to wake you up in the middle of the night when the alcohol levels in the blood are coming down. Avoid caffeine (in either coffee or tea) in the evening.

If you are awake at night it is helpful to have a technique to help you get back to sleep. You cannot make yourself go back to sleep but you can help to make yourself relaxed. Some people use a physical relaxation technique, either taking long slow breaths or tightening and then relaxing particular muscle groups. Sometimes these methods of relaxation require a good deal of movement and it can be difficult to fall asleep while you are doing them; however it can be a good way of quietening down the thinking processes. If you find you have a lot of thoughts going round and round in your head, you need to deliberately interrupt this, for example by saying in your mind: 'I won't go over this at the moment, I will focus on my relaxation technique.' If the thoughts come back again, try to follow the same process. You should not expect to be able to do this perfectly from the start but you should be trying to interrupt the thoughts at an earlier and earlier point.

The other technique to promote relaxation and sleep is a visualisation technique. Imagine that you are looking out at a scene that you know well and like – perhaps lying in a field looking at the crops and the trees beyond, with clouds floating by in a blue sky. Use these visualisations as a way of closing down the thoughts going round and round in your head. Some people take this technique to an extreme where they are looking at black to completely clear the mind – this can be very effective but is also very difficult to master.

These techniques need to be learned over time and it is usually easier to learn and get good at them when you are feeling well rather than when you are depressed.

3.39 How do I cope with suicidal thoughts?

Suicidal thoughts can either be distressing or quite comforting. The comforting aspect is thinking that suicide is an escape out of the mental pain and feeling that others will be relieved (or unburdened) if you are gone. Sometimes you can spend a lot of time thinking about exactly how you would commit suicide. Going through these plans, however, usually makes your mood worse. Like worrying, it is important to recognise when you are getting into this pattern and to try to interrupt your thinking. The other side of suicidal ideas is about the effect that your suicide would have on other people, as it is easy to let your negative thinking tell you that you do not matter. Try to remind yourself that periods of depression do pass and it is unusual to stay at the extremes of depression even when you suffer from severe manic depression.

3.40 How do I stop worrying?

It is also useful to have a general method of dealing with worries. The basic technique is to learn to recognise when you are worrying. Usually what happens is that you let the worries go round and round without recognising what you are doing, or the futility of these circulating thoughts. Worries are often about important things and so we feel that we need to think about them. However, there is a basic difference between worrying and thinking problems through – worrying just goes round and round and does not produce solutions. Often the problems you are worrying about have no solutions – for example they are about things that might happen. Recognise that the problem is worry rather than the subject of the worry!

3.41 What do I say to my friends and colleagues about my illness?

You need to judge this according to the person you are talking to. Many people will have very little understanding of manic depression and so you need to be wary about even using the term. There are a lot of assumptions and prejudices about manic depression that either are not true or don't apply in your case. When talking to most people it is reasonable to use the vaguest terms such as stress or depression. It is easier to do this than to tell them it is none of their business, even if it isn't their business! Do prepare an answer in advance and go through the scenario in your mind – you will feel much more confident if you have.

- 'Hello John, nice to see you back. I heard you were off sick, what's been the trouble?'
- 'Thanks for asking. Yes, I've been having a difficult time, got very stressed but I'm getting back on my feet now. How have things been in the office?'

An answer like this helps both you and your colleague to feel reasonably comfortable and you have moved the question onto neutral ground rather than leaving both of you with nothing to say at the end.

There are others who are more sympathetic or have had similar experiences, but manic depression is still uncommon so that friends may think that they understand what you have been through when they really don't. Using words like depression are probably appropriate in this case; however, be wary of talking too much about what has happened as friends may not be as interested as they appear and may also be quite judgemental. Often they will ask what they can do to help and try to have an answer to this, for example: 'What would be really useful would be if you could let me get on with the work on my own but then help me to check it to make sure that I'm doing OK.' This type of approach both acknowledges their sympathy and also ensures that what they are doing is helpful but not too intrusive.

Of course there are important people with whom you need to be completely honest – particularly your partner or a potential partner. If they haven't known you when you were unwell and you have made a good recovery then they will find it difficult to take on board the seriousness of your condition. This will take more than a few conversations, but the principles are the same as with others – try to tell them what is helpful for you and what dangers you need to avoid. It is easy to slip in with those who are minimising the seriousness of your illness as this is what you want to believe too!

Treatment of mania

4

4.1 What is the best treatment for mania?

The first step in the treatment of mania is to stop the antidepressants. There are then two main lines of treatment in acute manic relapses. The first is to increase the long-term treatment – for example if the patient is already taking lithium then the levels should be checked and, providing it is being tolerated reasonably well, to increase the dose, aiming for a level of up to 1.0 mmol/l (occasionally up to 1.2 mmol/l). A similar approach can be adopted with valproate and carbamazepine. The alternative line is to give a specific antimanic treatment, usually an antipsychotic, either on its own or in combination with a long-term treatment (*Fig. 4.1*).

4.2 How are antipsychotics used in mania?

The most commonly used medicines for the acute treatment of mania are the antipsychotic drugs (neuroleptics).

Until the introduction of the newer (atypical) neuroleptics the standard treatment was with haloperidol or chlorpromazine. These older treatments are effective but tend to cause a lot of side-effects, particularly parkinsonian symptoms such as tremor, shuffling and abnormal movements. They often cause akinesia and lack of facial expression but can also precipitate restlessness or akathisia where the patient has trouble sitting or standing still – a very distressing state. Akathisia can also be mistaken for the overactivity of mania. The main difference is that the manic patient likes being active but hates feeling restless, usually locating the restlessness of akathisia directly in their limbs rather than in their mind.

Traditional antipsychotics also have the advantage of being both sedative and calming which can be a considerable benefit in the early stages of treatment of mania. They still have a place in the emergency treatment of manic excitement and haloperidol (5 or 10 mg IM) is a safe drug to inject in these circumstances, usually in combination with procyclidine 10 mg to prevent dystonic reactions.

Olanzapine, quetiapine and risperidone are the atypical antipsychotics that are licensed for the treatment of mania but it is probably true that all antipsychotic drugs, including the newest one, aripiprazole, improve manic symptoms. These drugs are relatively free of parkinsonian side-effects, and are generally well tolerated (*Table 4.1*). They are available in either rapidly dispersing tablets or liquid which can be helpful when compliance is in doubt. Olanzapine is now also available as an injection.

The reason that antipsychotics are preferred to other medicines such as lithium and carbamazepine is that they are easy to use so an effective dose can be quickly reached. Additionally, most GPs are familiar with their use.

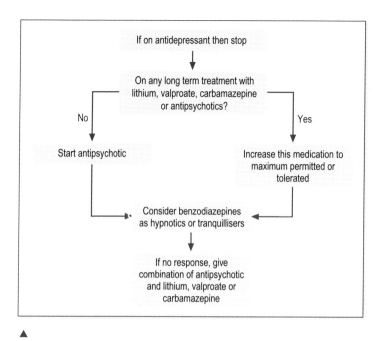

If on antidepressant then stop

On any long term treatment with
lithium, valproate, carbamazepine
or antipsychotics?

No   Yes

Start antipsychotic   Increase this medication to
                                                          maximum permitted or
                                                          tolerated

Consider benzodiazepines
as hypnotics or tranquillisers

If no response, give
combination of antipsychotic
and lithium, valproate or
carbamazepine

Fig. 4.1 Acute treatment of mania.

4.3   How quickly does antipsychotic treatment work?

Some improvement in manic symptoms should be seen within a few days of
starting the treatment (often due to a sedative effect), with a more substantial
recovery over 6 weeks. It is worth continuing one treatment line for 6 weeks
to assess response rather than changing or adding another treatment after a
couple of weeks. (This can require steady nerves since if there is no
improvement in the first 2 weeks everyone starts to wonder if you know what
you are doing!) If the level of activity or disturbance is high and sleeplessness
is a problem, prescribing benzodiazepines (diazepam or lorazepam) in
combination with the antipsychotics can be a useful short-term measure.

4.4   What other treatments are effective in mania apart from
antipsychotics?

VALPROATE

Valproate is the main alternative acute treatment and has the advantage of
being effective, well tolerated and easy to use. Depakote is the formulation

TABLE 4.1 Drugs used in the acute treatment of mania

Drug	Daily dose range (mg)	Most common side-effects	Comments
Haloperidol	5–20	Drowsiness, parkinsonism, dystonia	Can be given by injection; safe in a wide variety of doses
Chlorpromazine	50–500	As for haloperidol plus dry mouth	Very sedative
Olanzapine	10–20	Weight gain	Available in rapidly dispersing tablets and injection
Quetiapine	400–800	Sedation, postural hypotension	Usually well tolerated
Risperidone	2–6	Parkinsonism at higher doses	Available in liquid and in rapidly dispersing tablets

that is licensed for the treatment of mania as the studies have been done using this form (Bowden et al 2000, NICE Technology Appraisal 66). This particular formulation provides higher blood levels for the same apparent dose compared to other forms of valproate. The usual starting dose is 750 mg daily (250 mg tablets spread over two doses). It can then be increased gradually over a week up to 1500 mg or further to 2 g if necessary. It would seem likely that the other forms of valproate are also effective but licensed preparations are generally preferred (see National Institute for Clinical Excellence guidelines, www.nice.org.uk).

LITHIUM

Lithium is also an effective antimanic treatment and is used in similar doses and with similar blood levels to those used in preventive treatment (*see Chapter 5*). Higher doses with levels up to 1.0 mmol/l or even slightly higher than this are sometimes used. There are several difficulties in using lithium in mania:

■ Patients who are severely ill may be drinking little and are therefore liable to dehydration; this makes treatment with lithium more difficult and potentially dangerous.

■ It is difficult to find the effective dose rapidly as increases are usually done gradually: it can take a couple of weeks to reach a therapeutic dose and manic symptoms often need more urgent treatment than this.

■ Another reason relates to starting a long-term preventive treatment when a patient is manic and is not capable of making longer term decisions. Stopping lithium suddenly can cause a rebound manic effect (*see Chapter 5*). If lithium is started when patients are acutely manic and not committed to long-term treatment, they are likely to stop when they have recovered and this will risk precipitating a further episode of mania. This effect is not so apparent with antipsychotics and valproate.

For all these reasons antipsychotics or valproate are usually used first line; lithium is then added if the first line of treatment is not proving effective. In practice most patients are given a combination of treatment, with antipsychotics being added as an acute treatment to the longer term treatment, usually lithium.

CARBAMAZEPINE
Carbamazepine is also effective in the treatment of mania and it is useful to bear this in mind either as a primary treatment or increasing the dose if the patient is already on carbamazepine.

BENZODIAZEPINES
Benzodiazepines are also commonly used in mania. They are used generally for their sedative effect and particularly in cases where urgent calming and sleep induction are necessary. Lorazepam (0.5–1 mg) as an intramuscular injection is an effective emergency treatment for acute psychosis including mania (*see Q 4.9*). In the early days of treating excited manic patients many doctors give diazepam which has a long half-life, helps to improve sleep and has a calming effect during the day. Clonazepam is also used and there have been some studies to show this is effective in mania on its own, though it is unusual to treat mania only with benzodiazepines.

4.5 What if the mania is not improving on antimanic treatment?
This is a similar answer to that of treating depression that does not improve (*see Q 3.9*). The following questions should be considered before contemplating a change in medication:

- *Have you given the treatment long enough?*: For example, at least 4 weeks with no or only minor response. It can be difficult to stick with the treatment when there is little improvement, but if the treatment is changed too early the benefits of the medication may be missed.
- *Have you tried a higher dose?*: If the patient is not getting better, doses should be increased to the maximum dose that is recommended, provided that the treatment is reasonably tolerated before turning to an alternative antimanic.
- *Have you assessed concordance/compliance?*: This is usually a problem in the treatment of mania as most patients have limited insight into their condition and so are unlikely to be taking the treatment correctly. There is also a fair chance that they are deliberately concealing their

non-compliance rather than refusing. It is not uncommon to find a stack of tablets hidden away in a patient's room when they have appeared entirely willing to take the treatment (*see also Q 5.43*). Can you arrange some supervision of the treatment and give it in a formulation that is harder to evade – a liquid or dispersible tablet?

■ *Are they physically ill?* (*see Q 4.13*): Specifically, is their thyroid function normal?

■ *Have you got the diagnosis right?*: For example, is this really an episode of mania or is this a drug or alcohol problem?

■ *Is there another medication that they are taking that might be affecting their mania (e.g. steroids)?*

4.6 What are the next lines of treatment in mania that has not responded to the first antimanic treatment?

If the first line being followed is with a single medication then try a combination of treatments: an antipsychotic should be one medication together with another antimanic, usually lithium or valproate.

Although there are some reservations on using lithium in acute mania, if there is little improvement lithium must be considered and at a sufficient dose to give a level of about 1.0 mmol/l.

There are other options available but these would usually be restricted to specialist use. These include carbamazepine, lamotrigine (*see Q 3.4*), benzodiazepines (including clonazepam) or ECT (*see Q 3.22*).

4.7 How long should antimanic drugs be taken?

> The symptoms of mania need to have completely abated before considering slowly tapering off the antimanic medication.

As soon as the symptoms have begun to settle it is reasonable to start reducing the additional sedatives if these have been prescribed. If the patient is sedated by the antimanic treatment then this should also be cautiously reduced. These changes should be made slowly and on an experimental basis so that if symptoms re-emerge then the dose can be increased again.

Most doctors would wait 2–3 months after the manic symptoms have remitted to start slowly tapering the antimanic treatment, again watching for signs of relapse. This is the stage at which to have a discussion with the patient about longer term treatment.

4.8 How are psychotic symptoms in mania treated?

The antimanic treatments outlined above should lead to an improvement of psychotic symptoms as the other symptoms of mania abate. It is not essential to use antipsychotic medications when psychotic symptoms are present if other treatments (e.g. lithium or valproate) are being used. This differs from the advice in psychotic depression where antipsychotic drugs are always recommended. On the other hand mania without psychotic symptoms can be (and usually is) treated with antipsychotic drugs.

> The nomenclature of calling these drugs antipsychotics has never been satisfactory but 'neuroleptic' (the effect of making rats stop in their tracks) has never really caught on and the alternative of major tranquilliser is misleading as some of these drugs are not sedative. They are often referred to as dopamine antagonists, and this is almost certainly one of their most important pharmacological actions. However, they do have a number of other actions which are also likely to be important.

4.9 What treatment is useful in an emergency?

Acute manic excitement is a common psychiatric emergency which requires urgent sedation and calming. The usual treatment is with a sedative antipsychotic and a benzodiazepine. Oral medication is preferable unless the situation is so extreme that an injection is needed, either because rapid treatment is required or the patient is refusing or both.

> The standard emergency medication is haloperidol (5–10 mg IM), usually with procyclidine (10 mg IM or orally), along with lorazepam (0.5–1 mg IM). Similar doses can be used orally if the patient is willing to accept treatment.
> Now that olanzapine is available as an intramuscular injection (at a dose of 10 mg) this is likely to prove to be an effective and well-tolerated treatment in an emergency which can then be continued as an effective treatment for mania.
> It is important to look beyond the current crisis and ensure that effective antimanic medication is instituted to avoid returning a few hours later to deal with another emergency.

4.10 Do antipsychotics increase the risk of switching into depression?

One of the advantages of the newer (atypical) antipsychotics is that they do not have the mental clouding or dulling effect commonly described with haloperidol and chlorpromazine which can be mistaken for depression.

It is common for depression at some level to follow mania and about a third of patients can expect this. This may be in part an understandable reaction when the reality of the fallout from the manic behaviour is starting to impact. It is possible that antipsychotics exacerbate this tendency but if the patient is taking lithium then this medicine may help to prevent the depressive swing. Atypical antipsychotics may be less likely to precipitate depression.

In either case it is important to be on the lookout for depression and warn patients and their families about the possibility of post-mania depression. If this occurs it would increase the indication for longer term preventive treatment.

4.11 What treatment is effective for hypomania?

Hypomania – and this is partly in its definition – is a mild or even subclinical condition that may not require treatment in its own right. However, if patients are experiencing a series of depressive and hypomanic episodes then a trial of a long-term treatment (usually lithium or valproate) is the appropriate line.

If it is necessary to treat hypomania, the same lines of treatment as for mania should be followed. The difference in emphasis would be in favouring lithium or valproate rather than antipsychotics as almost invariably a long-term perspective needs to be taken since the condition is less severe in the acute phase.

It is important to consider whether antidepressants are exacerbating a bipolar II illness with more changes between depression and hypomania. If this is the case, antidepressant treatment is usually withdrawn (*see Q 6.23*).

4.12 Is ECT an effective treatment for mania?

Electroconvulsive therapy can be a useful treatment in mania though it is rarely used. It is reserved for those whose mania has become life-threatening because of nutritional or hydration problems and usually when other treatments are also being tried. The author has given it only once in the last 10 years and that was to a patient who had become almost impossible to communicate with and who wouldn't eat or drink although she gave no clear reason why not. The situation in which it is more commonly used is in the treatment of puerperal psychosis (*see Q 6.18*).

4.13 What investigations are needed?

The most important investigation is monitoring the physical state of the patient. Manic patients generally neglect themselves, in particular their nutrition and hydration. Sometimes they injure

> themselves through overactivity (e.g. their feet can become sore because they are walking so much, sometimes in bare feet). They may ignore minor injuries which can then become more complicated (e.g. by infection).

Apart from the general consideration of physical health, only simple blood tests are indicated. A full blood count may show an infection for which the patient had not mentioned any symptoms. Renal function is usually checked, particularly when lithium is being considered or dehydration is a concern. Checking liver function, particularly when mania is complicated by alcohol misuse, is also important. Most psychiatrists would also do a urine drug screen to ensure that other drugs (particularly stimulants such as amfetamines and cannabis) are not being taken. However, the most important investigations are repeatedly considering the physical state through simple observation and laboratory investigation.

There have been concerns that antipsychotics can have cardiotoxic effects (lengthening of the QT interval) and one of the newer antipsychotics (sertindole) was withdrawn because of this. A normal ECG can be reassuring, particularly when the QT interval is within normal limits. If high doses of drugs are being used, particularly in elderly patients, then an ECG should be routine.

4.14 How should I talk to a manic patient?

It can be time consuming, exasperating and exhausting talking to someone who is manic – rather than talking you need mostly to be listening! The patient will probably be rude, provocative, dismissive and abusive, and will almost certainly pick on a soft spot: how you are dressed, how you talk, anything the patient knows about you. Recognise that the patient is trying to wind you up rather than reacting to the provocation. Arguing back will only escalate the situation, though this is often hard to resist.

The patient may be joking with you, but be very careful about being jocular yourself as it often backfires.

Think what message you want to give the patient: the two most likely ones are about medicine and hospital. Try to give this message when you are given a chance, usually without much more explanation than 'It's because I think that you are ill'. Justify this in a basic way – for example 'You're not sleeping and you are getting agitated' – but it is rarely helpful to go into detail. Expect to repeat the message several times and try to stick with one line rather than letting the patient divert you.

Sometimes the patient will take up your offers while seeming to have very little insight. Giving a choice of medicine can sometimes be helpful so that it does not seem that the patient is giving in entirely to you.

Who does your patient trust, or who usually has some influence with them? Try to use this person as well, but be wary of putting such an individual in a difficult position; they may well prefer you to be making the decisions and they will probably already be very fraught, having been kept up all night anyway.

There is rarely a shortcut to getting manic patients to take some treatment, but with patience and persistence you can usually succeed. If not, you are likely to need to go down the route to detention in hospital.

If you are feeling rushed and trying to get away quickly you are very unlikely to make much progress!

4.15 How is the need for hospitalisation judged?

Making the decision to admit someone to hospital can be an easy one when the patient is very ill and putting themselves and others at risk. However, it can be a very difficult decision when the patient has only mild symptoms but is getting into difficulties in relationships and jeopardising their work. The decision about admitting someone into hospital is usually related to how effectively the family or other carers are able to cope with the patient and how cooperative the patient is with treatment.

When the illness is severe and the patient is psychotic then a period in hospital is very likely to be needed as the situation is very unpredictable. If there is violence or serious recklessness – particularly if they are driving – then the decision to admit is clear.

> In trying to predict what will happen in this manic episode, find out what happened in previous manias as this is the best guide. If there have been serious incidents of violence or reckless behaviour previously it makes sense to take preventive action and admit to hospital without waiting for this to happen again.

An agreement with the patient is desirable but this cannot be at the expense of ignoring potential dangers – the patient is likely to be minimising the problems and manic patients can be quite persuasive. This downplaying of the dangers, combined with the fact that this assessment will be time consuming and you are busy, can easily lead to decisions being made that on reflection don't seem quite so sound.

If hospitalisation isn't essential today, leave it open to review again tomorrow when it may be clearer. Take into account what the family says: the patient may well be behaving much better when you are there – manics can usually 'hold it together' for short periods of time and are likely to be doing so when the doctor calls!

Get an agreement about treatment and get this started. Checking if the patient is both saying they are willing to take the treatment and also putting this into action is a very important part of the assessment of whether they need to go into hospital. If they are not taking any treatment they will not get better in the near future.

The hardest judgement to make is how reckless does someone need to be to go into hospital. Is the fact that the person is irritable and annoying everyone sufficient reason? Probably not. But when does this cross over into seriously affecting relationships with family, neighbours and workmates which would be a good reason for taking someone out of this situation and into hospital? Likewise, seriously embarrassing behaviour by someone who is usually quiet and responsible can be very hard to live down and should prompt admission.

It is difficult to provide some of the benefits of hospitalisation at home. Being in hospital removes an individual from the social situation and if necessary the staff can stop patients from going out. This is usually impossible to reproduce at home even with frequent visits by community staff unless there is a very determined family. It is very unusual for someone who is manic to willingly stay put at home!

4.16 How is the need for compulsory detention for treatment in hospital judged?

The general assessment about hospitalisation is obviously relevant (*see Q 4.15*). However, if someone who is manic is not agreeable to going into hospital, then consider invoking legal powers (in England and Wales under the Mental Health Act 1983). The principles in most legal powers are:

1. *Does the person suffer from a mental illness?*: Are the usual symptoms of mania present and particularly does the person lack capacity to decide his or her own treatment? This is usually because of irrationality, either through psychosis or lack of insight. Can the individual recognise what is likely to happen if he or she does not have treatment or go into hospital?

2. *Is this illness so severe that it is justifiable to treat this person against their will?*: Would you feel justified in having this person admitted to a locked ward and given an injection forcibly which is a potential outcome of detention? You cannot detain someone only so far – detention means taking over responsibility from them.

3. *Are the risks so substantial in terms of their health and safety that there is no reasonable alternative?*: Have the alternatives been tried – for example getting the person to take the appropriate treatment voluntarily but found not to be possible? If the illness is not so severe but has been

continuing for several weeks without getting better despite everyone's best efforts, this may be another justification on health grounds.

If there is serious violence, people are getting hit or there is great recklessness (e.g. running down the middle of the road) then the decision to admit compulsorily is usually clear (*Case vignette 4.1*). Occasionally there may be a problem where the patient is not being violent though may be very provocative and irritating and someone else is hitting them!

CASE VIGNETTE 4.1 DISINHIBITION OF MANIA CAN LEAVE PATIENTS VERY VULNERABLE

Jane is a fourth year Modern Languages student. She suffered her first period of depression at the age of 17 while she was doing her A levels and had to defer a year because of this. She has had a difficult family background as her parents divorced when she was 10 and she has lived mainly with her mother ever since. Relationship between the parents has been particularly difficult and Jane's own relationship with her mother has always been strained.

She had a further episode of depression in her first year at university and was treated with a combination of an antidepressant (an SSRI) and a year of psychotherapy through the student counselling service. Early in her fourth year she had another period of depression which lasted about 4 months despite treatment with the same antidepressant which had seemed helpful before. This appears to have been a milder episode but more prolonged. Although she managed to continue with her studies, she was not doing as well as expected. She changed antidepressant to an SNRI and this seems to have been helpful. She made a reasonable recovery and is now studying effectively.

Suddenly the situation changes and a usually shy girl has gone off to Amsterdam and her parents are worried as she has texted her mum saying she is leaving university and is going to work in a bar in Amsterdam. Her father brings her back from Amsterdam in an excited, elated and over-talkative state. She thinks the time in Amsterdam has been fantastic but is also claiming that she has been raped. After a period in hospital she becomes depressed again and it is clear that she is very ashamed of her behaviour in Amsterdam where she had been promiscuous but then was raped by a man in the hostel she was staying in.

Periods of mania can lead not only to disinhibited behaviour but people can also put themselves at great risk of exploitation by others.

4.17 Can other specialist staff help in coping with a manic patient?

The mainstay of community psychiatry in the UK is the community psychiatric nurse (CPN). Experienced CPNs have usually had experience both in the hospital and the community so that they are familiar with a broad range of psychiatric problems and have also managed patients in extreme mental states. They often have a long-term relationship with both patients and their families which can prove invaluable in judging the seriousness of the mania and also what action is appropriate. CPNs are usually familiar with what medications have proved useful previously and how the illness tends to progress. In some cases they will be able to monitor the mental state on a daily basis and ensure that the medication is both available and ingested!

Social workers will need to be involved when compulsory detention is being considered, and will usually coordinate and organise this process, ensuring that the patient is admitted if they are detained. Social workers can also be helpful in providing practical help to families as well as patients.

Other members of the Community Mental Health Team include psychologists and occupational therapists. Their role is usually in the longer term care of people with manic depression (*see* Q 5.45). However these other team members can also be a useful resource in encouraging a manic patient to take some treatment, particularly if they have a strong relationship of trust with a patient or their family.

4.18 How often do patients commit serious crimes when they are manic?

It is surprising that manic patients do not feature more heavily in the statistics of psychiatric patients who have committed offences. One reason may be that they are so obviously ill that they are diverted from custody and being charged at a very early stage and so never reach court. Manic patients in hospital are often treated on intensive care units because of their intimidation and aggression and can be some of the most challenging patients to treat; however, it does seem that serious crimes of violence are rare. The fact that manics usually only become aggressive when they are thwarted may mean that violence is more common in hospital than outside. Other crimes, such as speeding and driving recklessly and dangerously, are much more common. It is always worth enquiring if your manic patients are driving as this is probably the most dangerous thing they are likely to do when manic.

4.19 Is violence a problem in mania?

Irritability is almost universally present in mania. It may not be apparent on first encounter, but as soon as the patient is thwarted or prevented from doing what is desired, then irritability will emerge.

The risk of violence is increased if there are other factors associated with aggression. The underlying personality and the person's usual propensity to use aggression is the main one. Those people who are usually peaceful and not liable to use violence to pursue arguments are unlikely to be violent when they are manic. Those who habitually favour aggression as the way to resolve problems are very likely to continue this when manic. The disinhibition of the illness and the confrontational situations that patients usually end up in will exacerbate this propensity.

Other aspects that need to be borne in mind when assessing violence in any situation are:

■ gender – males are the more violent sex
■ age – youth rather than the middle age
■ drug and alcohol misuse – reflecting both the direct disinhibiting effect and often the personality of the user.

4.20 What is the best way to deal with violent behaviour in a bipolar patient?

The first line is to assess the diagnosis and current clinical state. This can be a rapid process in a patient you know well and whose manic symptoms are obvious. If the patient is in an acute episode of mania but acting violently then urgent treatment including sedation is required (*see Q 4.9*). However, this can only be provided when the situation is safe – in hospital this is usually achieved using experienced and skilled staff in sufficient numbers to physically restrain the patient if this is necessary.

In the community, you have to use what resources are available, always remembering that your own safety is important. Calling the police is a sensible precaution when visiting a manic patient who has been reported to be violent or who has a history of violence. Sometimes knowing the patient well can actually make it easier to misjudge the situation. You will probably be used to seeing them when they are well and so consider them to be a generally reasonable person; however mania often leads to extreme behaviour which is completely unexpected. You may also think that you have a good relationship with the patient, but again this can go out of the window if the patient has become very irritable.

If you know that the patient has a weapon you should not approach – remember that knives kill and wound many more people than guns both in the UK and elsewhere.

If the situation is not that extreme and you decide it is reasonable to try to intervene, then the first step is to try to just talk – and more importantly listen – to the patient (*see also Q 4.14*). This gives you a chance to assess the patient's mental state and establish some rapport. Make sure you do not get into an argument – though this is very easy to do!

4.21 How do I resolve potentially violent situations involving bipolar patients?

Don't immediately try to resolve the situation – just listen and allow yourself to get some confidence in your diagnosis. You can only intervene in a medical way if this is a medical problem – bipolars get into arguments and violence for the same reasons as other people and this episode may not be a medical problem. Treat the person with interest and respect however rude they are.

Try to offer a solution:

- ■ *Would you like to come to hospital?*: It may seem unlikely that this will be accepted but it is worth offering none the less – it may offer a quick solution.
- ■ *Would you like to take some medicine to calm you down?*: Offer a choice of medicines (e.g. diazepam or olanzapine). It may be that if the patient has some control over the choice they would be willing to take some treatment – perhaps even ask them what medicine they think would be helpful.

It can be very time consuming coming to a resolution, and in dealing with the situation everything else will have to be dropped – a quick fix is unlikely to succeed. Use the other people around – who does the patient trust? Can they help to persuade the patient to have some medicine or go to hospital? However, make sure that others are not getting into arguments and winding the patient up; they are likely to be feeling very emotional in this situation and they have probably been dealing with it for hours or days already.

If you are not succeeding then the police may have to take over and they will probably have to use force to restrain the patient. If it comes to this you will have to make use of the Mental Health Act to deal legally with the situation. Usually when the formalities have been completed the patient will be taken by the police to hospital. Make sure that the hospital has a good (written) account of what has happened; it is invaluable to have a dispassionate account of what actual violence occurred. Was anyone injured? Were weapons used?

If anyone has been seriously injured then the patient will usually need to be detained in custody until a safe place (not an open acute psychiatric ward) is organised. It is the author's view that prosecution should be considered if any serious injury has occurred, but others think that if someone is ill this should not happen.

Afterwards, take care of yourself. These can be very frightening experiences, and if you have been hurt it can also leave you feeling very humiliated. We all react differently but talking about the experience, particularly with others who were involved, can be helpful. Avoidance increases anxiety – avoidance of the place, the people involved or even the thoughts all tend to make things worse rather than better.

4.22 What can family and friends do to help a manic patient?

There is a difficult balance to be struck when trying to help someone who is manic. The patient will almost certainly try to persuade you that they are fine and don't need any intervention. They often do this by a combination of cheerfully trying to get you to go along with them but also by getting irritable and annoyed if they are thwarted. Directly challenging patients often proves counterproductive but trying to make clear to them your view of their illness is important. Maintain your view that they are ill and what they need to do about it, without being drawn too much into argument.

It may take a lot of listening to get a chance to even make a simple point. Focusing on the practicalities is usually more productive than arguing about the principles which is often what happens. It is very time consuming dealing with people who are manic as they will talk endlessly to you and at you and productive dialogue is thin on the ground. You have to give them some time to speak but also to keep trying to draw them back to the important decisions that have to be made about their illness and its treatment. Some people are very skilful in edging patients along in a productive direction (e.g. taking treatment and medication) without it becoming a confrontation. This skill is more likely to be gained by experience rather than any particular techniques that can be learned. Do not get angry back as this is only rarely productive and usually escalates the situation.

4.23 Is an advance directive helpful when you are managing mania?

Having a good idea of what patients want you to do if they become ill again can be very valuable. An advanced directive is usually a written account of this (*see Appendix 2*). It will often include who should be involved – for example in the family, primary care or psychiatric staff. It may indicate what should be done about particular risks such as money, including taking away credit cards. The directive can specify what treatment the patient would prefer and hopefully this will have been worked out with a doctor beforehand.

There are plenty of positive uses for an advanced directive; however, they can still prove very difficult to implement. The patient may not accept at all what they have written down and on occasion it has been torn up in front of the doctor! The patient may well feel that it was someone else who really wrote it but felt under duress to agree; even so it gives you some basis to proceed with treatment. Some directives are unreasonably proscriptive – for example specifying who should be involved when they are either not available or not willing when the time arises. The treatment specified may not be appropriate and just because it is written down does not mean that it has to be implemented – you still have the usual responsibilities for your prescriptions. The directive may also specify that the patient does not wish to go to hospital or even that the illness should be allowed to continue its course – again you cannot ignore your responsibilities because of what is written down. If a patient is not capable of making decisions, then you have to act in their best interests, having taken account of all the relevant information that you have. In the end this may include detention through the usual legal channels.

Encourage patients to make advance directives and also encourage them to show them to people involved in their care, including the CPN and the family, so that everyone can have some input into their practicality.

 PATIENT QUESTIONS

4.24   How can I recognise that I am going manic?

It is often possible to identify a particular sequence of symptoms or behaviours that can act as a 'relapse signature' for each individual who experiences episodes of mania. Think back to what happened in the week or two before your illness became obvious. Look at the list of symptoms that occur in mania (*see Box 1.1*):

■ Do any of these symptoms occur early on in your illness?
■ Do you get particular ideas when you become manic – either grandiose or paranoid ideas or some very individual ideas (e.g. thinking that naturism should be universally adopted).
■ Ask other people what they notice early on that worries them (e.g. are you getting irritable or getting up very early to go running?).
■ Try to tie it to something measurable like sleep; if you are getting less than 6 hours something is probably going wrong.
■ Alternatively, think about what particular situations you get into with which people.

Write down your conclusions, or make a video so you can speak to yourself when you are manic, and decide in advance what you should do as it is difficult to make decisions when you are ill.

4.25   What can I do to help myself if I think that I am becoming manic?

All being well, you will have made a plan, even an 'advance directive', about what you should do in this circumstance. Try not to get annoyed when others are pressing you to implement the plan when you have lost insight. It is very easy when you are manic to find justifications for your behaviour and to blame others for the difficulties that you are running into.

Check out with your partner/friend/brother/sister whether they agree with you and what they think you should do.

Hopefully you will have agreed beforehand with your doctor what changes you will make to your treatment when you become manic. If you are on

PQ PATIENT QUESTIONS

longer term preventive treatment then it may be appropriate to increase this. Alternatively – and particularly if you are not on a long-term treatment – it will be starting an antipsychotic drug which suits you reasonably well and has been effective for you in the past. The short-term use of sleeping pills or tranquillisers might be another option.

Make sure you take good care of yourself. Eat decent meals, and above all make sure that you give yourself the opportunity to rest and particularly to sleep. Depriving yourself of sleep will definitely exacerbate your mania.

Should you stop going to work? Get someone else's advice on this as your judgement may not be good and it could be a big mistake turning up for work when you are disinhibited. Don't start drinking alcohol or smoking cannabis to calm yourself down as this will probably make things worse – intoxication increases disinhibition. Stop driving – its illegal to drive if you are not capable and driving is the most common way that people get seriously injured.

Get some advice from your doctor or nurse about what you should do. Go early so that they can confirm if you are taking the right action, and agree when you will review this again and what you should do if your symptoms get worse.

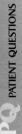

Lithium and long-term prophylactic treatment

LITHIUM

5.1 What is lithium?

Lithium is an element and in the same part of the periodic table as sodium and potassium. All of these elements are unstable and readily form salts. Lithium is found naturally in the form of lithium carbonate, which is dug out of the ground, mainly in Australia. There are good supplies throughout the world and provided that it is not all used up in a rush to make lithium-based batteries then there should not be a shortage in the foreseeable future.

5.2 How was lithium discovered?

John Cade, an Australian, is the doctor who is credited with introducing its modern use in psychiatry. In the 19th century, salts which included lithium were used for those suffering from mental illness, but this had not become accepted practice. Lithium had also been used as a diuretic and a salt substitute for those with cardiac failure earlier in the 20th century, but fell out of use because many patients ran into problems of toxicity. Cade was using lithium in an experiment on rats and thought that it had a calming effect on them and so a clinical trial in psychotic patients was undertaken. Lithium was found to be effective in the most active and agitated patients. Further studies in the 1960s and 1970s proved that it was an effective treatment for manic depression, though not without considerable initial scepticism.

5.3 How does lithium work?

We are not at all certain how lithium works. It is unlikely that it works directly on any neurotransmitter receptor in the brain, which is the putative mechanism of action of most psychotropic drugs (e.g. antipsychotics block dopamine receptors). Lithium tends to 'look like' calcium as a highly hydrated ion and may therefore affect the numerous actions of calcium on cells. The theory that is currently most popular is that lithium affects secondary messenger systems beyond the receptor including adenosine triphosphate (ATP) levels and G proteins.

5.4 How effective is lithium?

There are several ways to answer this question. Probably the simplest answer is that a third of patients who take lithium for manic depression have a very major, life changing benefit and their relapses are prevented, become much less frequent or much less severe. Another third will be likely to experience some benefit and notice a reduction in the severity or frequency of their illness, but still be experiencing significant symptoms. The other third really gain very little benefit from treatment with lithium and alternatives need to be considered (Prien et al 1973, Quitkin et al 1981).

The more statistical view of group effects is that lithium will reduce the rate of relapse by 20–30% (*Fig. 5.1*). The relapse rates in most trials are about 50% over a year on placebo and this is reduced to about 30% on lithium. However, it is difficult to translate this figure to individuals.

5.5 What are the indications for lithium treatment?

The most common reason for prescribing lithium is as a prophylactic treatment in bipolar illness. Lithium is more usually used for the prevention of bipolar illness with mania rather than hypomania though it is effective in both disorders. It is also effective in the treatment of mania and bipolar depression. It can be used on its own for the treatment of bipolar depression but is more commonly prescribed in combination with an antidepressant.

Lithium is also useful in the acute treatment of unipolar depression in combination with an antidepressant. Lithium is usually prescribed for those patients who are suffering from depression but have had only a partial response to an antidepressant; lithium is added to augment this treatment. It is the only well-validated augmenting strategy for unipolar depression (Anderson et al 2000, Goodwin 2003). Lithium also has a place in the prevention of recurrent unipolar depression.

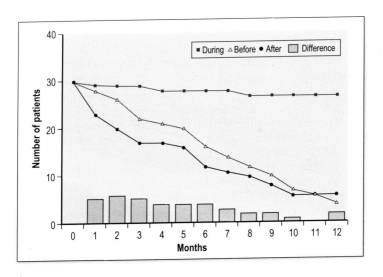

▲
Fig. 5.1 Lithium reduces the relapse rate in manic depression; stopping lithium precipitates relapse, beyond natural history. (Based on data from Schou 1993.)

Lithium is occasionally prescribed for certain forms of headache (e.g. cluster headaches).

Lithium has also been tried in a number of other disorders but no method of treatment is proven – for example it has been tried as a way of reducing aggression in those with a learning disability or helping alcoholics to reduce their intake or prevent relapse.

5.6 Who should be taking long-term preventive treatment for bipolar disorder?

If someone has had even a single, severe, highly disruptive episode of mania or severe depression then it is tempting to suggest that they should take long-term treatment and indeed a few patients do this. However, after one episode it is very uncertain when the next episode will occur (though it almost certainly will occur at some time, *see Q 2.18*) and most people will not want to undertake a very long-term treatment at this stage.

For those who experience a recurrent bipolar illness the decision to take long-term treatment is based on the frequency of relapse, the severity and length of episodes and the impact of the illness on normal life.

One estimate is that if someone has just recovered from an episode of illness and had a previous one in the last 4 years, then that person should probably take a preventive treatment. This is based on the expectation that lithium will be likely to prevent at least one major relapse over the next 5 years.

5.7 What are the common side-effects of lithium treatment?

Most people taking lithium should expect to experience an increase in thirst and, accompanying this, an increase in frequency of urine. Often when patients initially start treatment they experience a diuresis.

The other common symptom is tremor which is an exaggeration of the normal essential tremor. It is very likely that patients will experience these two side-effects but usually at a mild level.

Another side-effect which is commonly reported is weight gain. It is difficult to know why patients gain weight. For some it is clearly related to them drinking a lot of sweet fluids which appear to slake the thirst better than water. In others the cause is rather obscure and they tend to gain weight even though they don't feel that they are eating or drinking any more.

Many patients with manic depression, both when they are taking lithium and when they are not, complain of concentration and memory problems. It is not clear if lithium at therapeutic levels causes cognitive problems. Depression even at a low level can also affect cognition and disentangling these effects for individual patients is difficult.

5.8   Can lithium have long-term harmful effects?

The two major concerns about long-term lithium treatment are permanent effects on the thyroid and kidney. Hypothyroidism occurs in about 10% of those who take lithium and will usually persist even if the lithium is stopped.

Lithium can also affect the ability of the body to concentrate urine, which is the mechanism behind the excessive thirst and drinking that many patients experience. The biochemical explanation is that the kidney is not responsive to antidiuretic hormone (ADH). This effect usually reverses when lithium is stopped but can occasionally be persistent. There should be no permanent damage to the kidney if there are no episodes of lithium toxicity.

5.9   How dangerous is it?

Lithium poisoning through very high blood levels (3 mmol/l and higher) can cause permanent damage to the brain and kidneys and is potentially fatal. Damage to the brain often affects the cerebellum in particular and can leave patients permanently disabled. Likewise renal function can be permanently compromised by toxicity.

However, when the levels are kept below 1.2 mmol/l then lithium is very unlikely to cause long-term harmful effects on either the brain or the kidney. Usually those that suffer from toxicity do so because the levels have slowly gone up rather than in an acute overdose. Although lithium is obviously known to be dangerous at high levels it is surprising how rare overdoses of lithium seem to be, especially given that it is prescribed to a group that is exceptionally vulnerable to suicide (*see Q 5.26*). This may be because it is a very effective treatment and also that it may have a specific antisuicidal effect. However, the most serious adverse effects of lithium toxicity do seem to occur among those who deliberately take a large overdose of slow release tablets where the levels continue to rise long after ingestion even if they have vomited.

5.10   What are the symptoms of lithium toxicity?

As the blood level rises above 1.5 mmol/l people start to feel generally physically unwell, go off their food, feel nauseous and may start to vomit. They will also be likely to experience diarrhoea. In fact gastro-intestinal symptoms are very useful warning symptoms of impending toxicity. As the blood level continues to rise above 2.0–3.0 mmol/l neurological symptoms appear with stiffness, ataxia and confusion. If the levels continue to rise confusion becomes more prominent and coma, cardiovascular collapse and convulsions will appear.

Levels can reach as high as 5.0 mmol/l and fatalities and permanent physical damage can be expected.

It is important that patients know the early symptoms of toxicity, particularly the gastrointestinal ones, so that if they do experience these symptoms they can take action early. Obviously a lot of people experience occasional diarrhoea and vomiting from food poisoning but consideration that this may be a symptom of lithium toxicity is important.

However, the levels can be quite confusing, as patients can still have prominent symptoms of toxicity even though the serum level is no longer high. This is because the lithium level in the tissues is still high.

5.11 What are the common reasons for patients becoming toxic?

Toxicity often creeps up on patients rather than suddenly hitting them. This can be because there is a gradual decrease in renal clearance with age and if the lithium levels are not monitored regularly the level can slowly increase with only a gradual onset of warning symptoms. Iatrogenic factors are also important and the commonest reason for toxicity is the addition of a thiazide diuretic to lithium treatment. This reduces clearance of lithium and toxicity follows.

Other commonly prescribed drugs that can interact with lithium to increase levels are non-steroidal anti-inflammatory drugs such as ibuprofen and so particular care needs to be taken when treating bipolar patients who also have arthritis.

It is important to warn patients that they must check that any medicines they are going to take are compatible with lithium.

5.12 What needs to be done prior to initiating lithium treatment?

The most important test is to ensure that renal function is normal. In physically healthy patients this can be done by checking their creatinine levels; in those whose renal function is impaired or likely to be impaired (e.g. the elderly) it is necessary to do a creatinine clearance test. Lithium can affect thyroid function (and abnormal thyroid function can also affect the course of bipolar illness) so checking thyroid function prior to initiation is also necessary.

Ensure that the patient has been given a leaflet outlining lithium treatment (*see model in Appendix 3*) as they will not remember enough from a conversation. Stress the symptoms of toxicity that need to be recognised, and also that careful use of lithium and good monitoring will prevent toxicity occurring. An example of specific instructions from the hospital about how to start treatment are shown in *Figure 5.2*.

Dear Dr Henderson

RE: Mr M Depression – 09.06.57
8 Serenity Drive, Shelford, Cambs CB2 5EF

I saw Michael again this week, his wife came with him this time and she confirmed the pattern of his manic depressive illness. I understand that Michael has also been in to discuss further treatment with you.

We agreed that he will now have a trial of lithium treatment. We discussed this and in particular the need to be vigilant for symptoms of toxicity such as vomiting and diarrhoea and the importance of not stopping the lithium suddenly because of a manic rebound. He has already looked at the leaflet about this treatment that I gave him last time.

I understand that he has had the blood tests now and that his renal and thyroid functions are normal, therefore he could start lithium carbonate (Priadel) 400 mg at night and will get his first lithium level checked after 5–7 days. We discussed the need to take the lithium at night so that a level could be taken in the morning, 12 hours after taking the tablet.

If this level is lower than 0.6 he should increase up to 600 mg at night and I will review this with him 2 weeks after starting lithium.

I hope you are in agreement with this line of treatment and if you would like to discuss this, do feel free to call me.

With best wishes
Yours sincerely

Copy to: Mr M Depression

▲

Fig. 5.2 Example of a letter from a consultant to both GP and patient about starting lithium treatment.

The other important piece of information the patient should know is that this is a long-term treatment and sudden cessation of lithium can lead to rebound mania and so a worsening of the illness course (*see Q 5.27*). This means that the illness can be made worse by taking lithium intermittently than it would have been if the patient had never taken the treatment at all!

5.13 How is lithium treatment initiated?

Assuming that preliminary checks have been made (*see Q 5.12*) and renal function is normal, the usual routine for beginning lithium treatment would be to start at 400 mg at night and then check a blood lithium level at 5 days. It is likely that the initial target blood level will be 0.6 mmol/l and benefit will be judged at this level. If the blood level at 5 days comes back at less than 0.6 mmol/l the lithium dosage should be increased by 200 mg and checked again at 5 days. This process should be repeated until the desired level is reached. When a stable dose has been reached, continue to monitor every 2 weeks for 1 month, then monthly for a further 3 months and 3-monthly thereafter.

5.14 Why is lithium usually prescribed to be taken all at night?

There is no good therapeutic reason for taking lithium at night – it is no more effective then than if taken at any other time. However, side-effects are generally more prominent at higher blood levels which tend to be in the first few hours after taking the tablet (*see Fig. 5.3*), so it can be preferable for the patient to be asleep at this time. For compliance reasons taking tablets once a day is usually better (*see Q 5.43*).

However, the main issue is arranging serum lithium estimations. These need to be taken 12 hours after the last dose so that if the lithium is taken in the evening it is relatively easy and convenient to do a blood test the following morning. The alternative of taking the tablets in the morning and doing blood tests in the evening causes not only logistic problems but also often results in samples being kept overnight which can affect other blood tests (e.g. potassium levels) that are done at the same time.

Some people find that splitting the doses of lithium between morning and evening is preferable, usually because this can reduce side-effects. This can make monitoring confusing if a blood test is taken only a couple of hours after the last dose which shows a high (peak) level. Patients should be asked to delay the morning dose until after the blood test, so that a trough level is measured.

5.15 What formulation of lithium should be prescribed?

Lithium is the same whatever formulation it comes in – tablets, slow release versions or liquid – carbonate or citrate. However, the dose is not interchangeable between different formulations and one cause of toxicity is a change of formulation. Different formulations have different bioavailabilities and if the formulation is changed then move to a lower dose and then monitor on a weekly basis until the levels are stable. The most common reason for doing this is changing to a liquid if the patient is not getting on well with tablets, as they are large tablets which can be difficult to swallow.

Currently in the UK lithium carbonate (Priadel) is the most commonly prescribed tablet. It is probably a good idea for all the patients in a practice to be taking the same formulation to reduce the possibility of prescribing errors.

5.16 What monitoring needs to take place while on lithium treatment?

When the patient is on a stable dose of lithium, checking lithium levels every 3 months is adequate; checking renal and thyroid function every year is also needed. Weight gain can be a problem with lithium and keeping an eye on this from the start rather than waiting until the patient has gained weight is worthwhile. There have been reports of hyperparathyroidism with lithium and some advocate checking calcium levels annually as well (Drug and Therapeutics Bulletin 1999).

5.17 Are lithium cards useful?

It is very helpful if patients keep a note of all their blood tests, so that whichever doctor they see there is a readily available record. This needs to include doses of drugs, dates of lithium levels, and also renal and thyroid function, thus allowing blood tests done either in the hospital or in general practice to be easily accessed.

Some pharmacies and clinics give out cards that are marked up to include spaces for the range of monitoring that is needed. Sometimes patients keep a notebook with various details about their treatment; no doubt some now use electronic means!

5.18 What blood levels should I be aiming for?

The therapeutic range that is routinely aimed for is 0.4–0.8 mmol/l in the serum at 12 hours after the last dose (*Fig. 5.3*). When lithium was first introduced into psychiatry, higher levels of up to 1.2 mmol/l were commonly used but over the years the level aimed for has tended to be lower. This is probably because doctors have become more concerned about toxicity, even though with care higher levels can be maintained safely.

Levels need to be at least 0.4 mmol/l in order for lithium to be an effective treatment, and no patient should be maintained below 0.4 mmol/l.

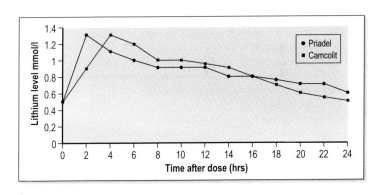

Fig. 5.3 Daily variation in lithium level. (Based on data from Bennie et al 1977.)

Even levels of 0.4 mmol/l may not be enough and the usual practice would be to aim for a level of between 0.6 and 0.8 mmol/l. If this is not well tolerated a trial at lower levels down to 0.4 mmol/l is reasonable. If lithium is well tolerated at levels between 0.6 and 0.8 mmol/l but is only partially relieving or preventing symptoms, then higher levels up to 1.0 mmol/l (or even up to 1.2 mmol/l in acute treatment) may be needed and can be safely used with appropriate monitoring.

5.19 How should I react to a high blood lithium level?

If a lithium level comes back between 1.0 and 2.0 mmol/l it is important to consider the possible reasons for this and to ascertain the patient's physical and mental state. Often higher readings come back because the blood sample has been taken less than 12 hours after the last dose (*see Fig. 5.3*). This may be because the patient is taking the lithium in the morning and has had a blood test only a few hours later. It is important to establish first whether this might be the case.

Next: How is the patient? The clinical assessment is more important than the blood level as patients can be toxic at apparently regular levels (<1.0 mmol/l) and not toxic at apparently high levels well over 1.0 mmol/l. If the patient has no symptoms of toxicity and seems well otherwise it is usually safe to continue on the lithium and have another estimation of the lithium level, aiming for as accurately at 12 hours after the last dose as possible. However, if there are symptoms of lithium toxicity (e.g. diarrhoea and vomiting) it is necessary to stop the lithium temporarily and then take another level. If the level is only marginally high (e.g. 1.0 mmol/l when the usual level is 0.8 mmol/l) and there are only mild changes (e.g. loose stools but not vomiting or neurological symptoms) then a reduction of the dose and a further blood test may be appropriate.

If the patient has prominent neurological symptoms (including confusion) or cardiovascular symptoms this would indicate the need for hospital admission. The usual treatment is intravenous infusion of normal saline but very high levels (e.g. 4.0 mmol/l) will be likely to require dialysis.

Overall, the level of symptoms, together with the clinical assessment, is more important than the blood levels. It is easy to keep changing the lithium dose frequently in response to blood levels but then to find it difficult to reach a stable dose. It is generally better to re-check levels rather than changing doses if there are no symptoms of toxicity. Dose changes in long-term treatment should be made only if two or three levels indicate the need for this (*see Case vignette 5.1*) unless there are symptoms of toxicity or the clinical state requires it.

5.20 How should levels above the usual therapeutic range be dealt with?

Case vignette 5.1 illustrates the difficult balance that needs to be made between clinical state, side-effects, lithium level and dose. Sometimes it is difficult to understand what is happening but the focus on the physical side-effects, mental state and the timing of the levels is the main guide to treatment. Even high levels do not immediately lead to a change in dose, but if the clinical state is satisfactory then a repeat level is the appropriate action.

Having a good degree of concordance with the patient described in *Case vignette 5.1* about treatment and monitoring, along with her giving a high value to the benefit of lithium in treating the depression (because of the severity of the symptoms prior to treatment) enabled us to persevere with this treatment when other patients may have decided to try an alternative, even though the potential benefits would be uncertain.

CASE VIGNETTE 5.1 BALANCING LITHIUM LEVELS

A woman in her forties has a history of hypomania but has now had chronic depression for more than a year which has prevented her from working though she has maintained basic domestic tasks. Treatment with amitriptyline up to 225 mg daily has led to only partial improvement but there has been no recurrence of manic symptoms. It is agreed to add lithium to the antidepressant because of the need to augment the antidepressant treatment and also to prevent recurrence of hypomania. Her renal and thyroid functions are normal.

She reaches stable levels of 0.6–0.7 mmol/l on a dose of 600 mg and there is a substantial improvement in her depression over 6 months. However, there are occasional levels that are higher (e.g. 1.2 mmol/l) but further investigation shows that this was a 10 hour level when she usually gets levels at 14 hours.

However, her depressive symptoms then worsen and the dose is increased to 800 mg. The levels increase to 0.9–1.1 mmol/l. She has some tremor and thirst but the improvement in depression is more than compensating for this. One level is as high as 1.2 mmol/l but her side-effects are not worse and she continues on 800 mg; on repeat testing the level has dropped to 0.9 mmol/l.

However, 3 months later she develops diarrhoea and her level is measured at 1.2 mmol/l. Because the physical symptoms are more prominent the dose is decreased to 600 mg. The level drops to 0.6 mmol/l on the two follow-up samples over the next 2 weeks, and the diarrhoea resolves. Her depressive symptoms become more prominent and so an increase is made in the lithium to 700 mg (levels of 0.8 and 0.9 mmol/l) and then to 800 mg. However, the levels now go up to 1.5 mmol/l, though again this is at 10 hours. Because she has prominent tremor and thirst the lithium dose is reduced to 700 mg and levels of 0.9 mmol/l are then maintained.

5.21 Is there a lack of lithium in the blood of manic depressives?

No, everyone has a trace of lithium in their body and we probably all need a tiny daily intake of lithium, as we do with many other trace elements which we get from our food. However the amount of lithium needed is about 1 mg a day whereas the smallest tablet of lithium is a hundred times more than this. Those who have manic depression are no different from anyone else in the amount of lithium they naturally have in their body.

Sometimes patients see lithium treatment as 'correcting a chemical imbalance'. It is often unclear exactly what they mean by this although it is likely that there are some neurotransmitter changes in the brain of a person who is manic or depressed. It is possible that these changes reverse with effective treatment and so lithium is 'correcting an imbalance'. However, the chemical imbalance is not a constitutional lack of lithium. These phrases are often used as useful metaphors that can be agreed with the patient even if neither of you actually knows clearly what the other means!

5.22 What effect does lithium have on the developing foetus?

There is a definite risk of abnormalities in the foetus when the mother has been taking lithium during the pregnancy. This is an effect in the developmental part of the pregnancy, i.e. the first trimester. The best recognised abnormality is Ebstein's anomaly, which is a severe and potentially fatal cardiac abnormality. However, the relationship of this to lithium has been questioned in recent years.

The risk of any congenital abnormality in 'normal' pregnancies is about 3% and in those taking lithium about 11%. This means that the great majority of babies will not have any recognisable abnormality, but this level of congenital abnormality is not usually an acceptable risk for mothers to take.

Similar levels of abnormalities have been recorded in the offspring of women who have taken carbamazepine or valproate (though most research has been done in those with epilepsy, not manic depression); neural tube defects appear to be the highest risk. Folate supplementation is recommended for all women planning pregnancy (400 mcg daily before conception and during the first 12 weeks of pregnancy) and is particularly advocated for women taking these drugs.

Apart from congenital abnormalities which occur in the first trimester, the effects on the foetus in the latter part of pregnancy can also be significant (e.g. on the thyroid or heart rhythm) and there may still be some risk in taking lithium even at this stage.

Balancing the risks of medications and the risk of relapse if the treatment is stopped is an exceptionally difficult decision that can only be made on an individual basis (*see Q 5.25*).

5.23 What is the management for a bipolar woman who has been successfully treated with lithium but now wants to become pregnant?

Decisions around treatment of bipolar women in regard to reproduction is an exceptionally difficult area and expert advice is needed. Several factors need to be balanced.

1. There are small but definite risks of lithium to the foetus (*see Q 5.22*). A judgement needs to be made whether it would be possible for the potential mother to come off lithium and remain well off this treatment prior to becoming pregnant. This might be possible for a woman who has been stable for several years where the risk of relapse is judged to be low. Unfortunately the common scenario is that when you try to slowly reduce the lithium she experiences a relapse and you are back to where you started. Some women opt to continue with the lithium while they become pregnant even knowing the risks to the baby and then ensure that the pregnancy is closely monitored and the foetus assessed for abnormalities at an early stage.
2. An alternative is to try a different medication during pregnancy. Older antipsychotic drugs such as chlorpromazine may be effective in the prevention of mania and are not thought to carry an increased risk of foetal abnormality. This is a possible option during pregnancy instead of lithium. Treatment with alternative preventive medications, particularly the anticonvulsants carbamazepine and valproate, run similar overall risks of malformation (though the particular malformations are different) to the growing baby.
3. The immediate postpartum period is an exceptionally vulnerable time for women and there is about a one in three chance of relapse, mania being more common than depression postpartum. Most doctors would recommend that if the woman has gone through pregnancy without lithium that she restarts this treatment immediately after childbirth and not breast feed.

5.24 Is it appropriate to breast feed while taking lithium?

No. There would have to be a very good reason why women are feeding their babies in this way if they are taking lithium as there is a substantial chance that the baby will experience toxic symptoms.

5.25 For how long should a bipolar patient continue to take lithium?

The first goal of any long-term treatment is to judge whether the drug is acceptable. Some patients are particularly sensitive to lithium and cannot take it even at therapeutic levels. For example a female bipolar patient found that she was getting diarrhoea even at levels of 0.4 mmol/l and so could not continue with a trial of treatment for longer than a month.

If the treatment is acceptable and reasonably tolerated then the next aim is to judge whether lithium is beneficial. This usually needs to be done over 6 months to 1 year, so that even if the patient suffers a relapse in the first few months it is usually worth continuing the treatment to make a longer term judgement as to whether lithium is providing a reduction in severity or frequency of relapse compared to the period prior to taking it. There is also a judgement to be made of balancing efficacy against tolerability.

If lithium does prove beneficial it needs to be taken long term. The propensity to recurrence in manic depression never goes away and if someone is doing well while on lithium there needs to be a very good reason to stop it. The experience of seeing a patient who has been well for 10 years or more while on lithium and then deciding to stop it and rapidly experiencing a relapse is not uncommon (*Case vignette 5.2*).

Statistically the time needed to prevent a relapse is 1–2 years so that patients who take lithium for a shorter period may be getting no benefit from it and if they stop it suddenly may well be making their illness worse through rebound effects. Taking the treatment for 6 months and suddenly stopping may mean that the illness course is worse than never having taken it at all. (*see Q 5.27*).

It is worthwhile discussing with patients that if lithium is beneficial they should continue taking it unless there is a very good reason to stop. Some patients may ask if they are taking it for life – a reasonable response is that they should be taking it for several years but with review as to how they are, how helpful the treatment is, what problems they are getting with the medicine and then make a decision as to whether to continue. There may, of course, be other treatments that emerge in the coming years which will replace lithium or indeed provide a permanent cure – but currently lithium is still the treatment most likely to be of benefit to manic depressives.

CASE VIGNETTE 5.2 STOPPING LITHIUM SUDDENLY

Peter was ill as a student (probably mania followed by depression), reading law at university. His father took him away for an extended holiday in Spain where he built walls, as Churchill had recommended. He got back to university and then qualified as a barrister. He had been brought up abroad and returned to Uganda to work and built up a sound legal practice. However, the arrival of Idi Amin put paid to that and he returned to England in a very depressed state from which he took a year to recover. He then worked in the Caribbean as a government lawyer for 10 years but this ended when he became manic, spent all his savings on yachts and was sacked. A further period of depression back home in England with family followed and he then moved to Australia. This was the first time that he had been prescribed lithium and his wife ensured that he took it every night. He worked successfully for 15 years and restored his affluent lifestyle. He had a talk with his doctor about the lithium and they both decided that he had been well for a long time and could reasonably give it up now. Within a month he had redecorated and re-carpeted his office in yellow. He attended court, not in his usual sober suit, but in a tee-shirt with a cork hanging hat. He was quickly suspended and flew off to Penang first class to gamble, drink and carouse. He was arrested and deported for not paying his hotel bill. On return to Australia he was committed to hospital, for which he never forgave his wife and they separated. He lost his job, his home and his wife and still lives in a hostel near the beach – he has started to take the lithium again.

5.26 Does lithium really reduce the rate of suicide?

There are two reasons why we think that lithium prevents suicides:

1. Lithium is effective in reducing the burden of illness in manic depression by both treating and preventing mania and depression. A reduction in the frequency and severity of depression would be likely to reduce the rate of suicidal acts.
2. There may be a specific effect of lithium on reducing suicidal thoughts and impulses which is why it has been tried in other groups who are known to be suicidal (e.g. those who frequently self-harm such as those with borderline personality disorder).

The research on non-bipolars is unclear. Anecdotally lithium does seem to be effective for some patients but many doctors feel it is very risky giving a medication which is known to be very dangerous in overdose to patients who regularly take overdoses!

Even among bipolars it is difficult to interpret the studies which indicate that the suicide risk is much lower on lithium. The patients in these studies who are most compliant and reliable in taking lithium may also be those who are least likely among the manic depressives to be impulsive and suicidal, so that comparison of those on and off lithium is not comparing like with like. However, post mortem inquiries into patients with manic depression who have committed suicide show that they are unlikely to have been taking or even been prescribed lithium. Overall, it is likely that lithium does have a strong benefit in reducing the risk of suicide if it is taken in the long term (Schou 1998).

5.27 Does stopping lithium suddenly lead to relapse?

Probably the best way to make bipolar patients manic is to treat them with lithium for a few months then suddenly stop it. About a third of patients will relapse, usually into mania rather than depression, in the following few weeks (*Fig. 5.4*). This is a rebound effect in that patients do not return to the underlying natural history of manic depression but 'rebound' beyond this to a much higher chance of recurrence.

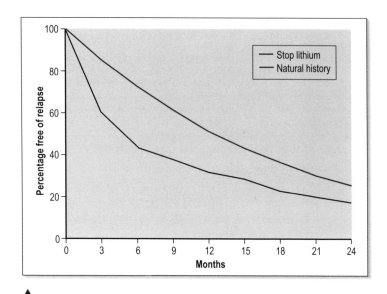

▲

Fig. 5.4 Sudden lithium withdrawal causes rapid relapse in bipolar disorder (usually into mania). (Based on data from Suppes et al 1991.)

If lithium is stopped gradually over 4–6 weeks then the risk of relapse is less than with sudden cessation and patients return to the risk associated with the natural history and avoid the rebound. However, many doctors would stop the treatment even more slowly, so that any emerging symptoms can be responded to by increasing the dose of lithium again.

If a patient is well on lithium there needs to be a very good reason for stopping treatment – manic depression does not go away. If the patient is well it is likely that this is because the treatment is working effectively. There is a strange paradox in the treatment of many medical conditions in that those who are doing worst (and presumably getting the least benefit from the treatment) are those that we most encourage to continue and take higher doses, whereas those who are well (and presumably getting the most benefit) are often encouraged (or not discouraged) to stop (*see Case vignette 5.2*)

5.28 If the patient stops lithium and suffers a relapse, does it work as well the second time around?

There has been concern that the effect of lithium is reduced when it has been stopped suddenly and a relapse has occurred. This is a difficult question to answer as we know that the more episodes a patient has, and the shorter the well interval, the worse the prognosis. If a patient had an extra episode through stopping lithium then their prospects over the next year would be less good than if they had avoided this relapse. However, if there has previously been a good response to lithium then it is definitely worth going back to this treatment again after a relapse, and not shifting on principle to a different medication.

5.29 Why do manic depressives who are doing well on lithium stop taking it?

Doctors usually expect that the main reason that patients stop taking medications is either because the treatment is not effective or that side-effects are unacceptable. Given that everyone on lithium can expect to experience some side-effects and treatment is only partially effective, the assumption is that this is why some patients stop. However, the common scenario is of a bipolar patient who is doing well on the treatment and having only minor side-effects deciding to stop because he does not think that he is going to be ill again. It is very hard for patients to accept that they have little control over their mood and that even if they have their life on track and no serious stressors, they are still liable to a recurrence. It is common to hear comments such as: 'When I got ill before I was having particular problems at work and I've sorted them out now, so I just don't think it will happen again.' It may well be true that they are helping to protect themselves by sorting out the problems at work but it is likely that it is not sufficient to prevent a relapse.

Of course the usual reasons (lack of efficacy and side-effects) apply not only to lithium but also to other long-term treatments and there are other associations with non-compliance (*see Q 5.43*) including personality factors and substance misuse.

5.30 Are there particular illness patterns which are likely to improve with treatment?

Finding patients who are particularly likely to benefit from treatment with lithium is not generally possible. Family history can be useful; if you know that someone else in the family has done well with lithium then it would in all probability be beneficial to move the patient to this treatment sooner rather than later. The pattern of illness – mania into depression and then recovery – is thought to be a pattern particularly responsive to treatment with lithium.

OTHER LONG-TERM TREATMENTS

5.31 Is valproate a useful long-term treatment in bipolar illness?

Mania can be effectively treated with valproate (*see Q 4.4*). It relieves the symptoms of mania as effectively as any other treatment and because it is generally well tolerated the dose can be increased rapidly even in patients who have never taken it before. Valproate may be the best treatment to give to those who are in a mixed episode (a simultaneous combination of mania and depression – *see* Q 1.11).

Many patients are treated with valproate as a long-term preventive measure. However, it is much less certain if this is an effective treatment and as the evidence currently stands it should not be given as a first line preventive treatment. On the other hand, it should be considered in those who are unresponsive to lithium and may be more effective than lithium in those who are in a rapid cycling phase of the illness. The doses needed for long-term treatment are similar to those used in the acute treatment of mania, but it is usually introduced more slowly as the clinical situation is usually less urgent. The medication is usually started at 200 mg twice a day and increased gradually over a month to 1200 mg/day. Sometimes higher doses of up to 2 g/day are needed. Although it is recommended that it is taken twice a day this can limit compliance and for those who have great difficulty in taking it this often, consideration should be given to prescribing it all in one dose of a slow-release version of valproate.

5.32 Are there any problems with taking valproate?

 Valproate is generally a well-tolerated drug. The only common side-effects are gastrointestinal with nausea and occasionally vomiting. Less common side-effects are neurological with tremor and unsteadiness. Rarely it can cause liver dysfunction, though this seems to occur mainly in children, and also rarely pancreatitis.

5.33 Is there a difference between sodium valproate and valproate semi-sodium (Depakote)?

The basic drug in these two formulations is the same: the semi-sodium formulation (Depakote) is a combination of valproic acid with sodium valproate, hence the semi- or half-sodium. It is absorbed as a combined molecule and later broken up into valproate. Virtually all of the trials of valproate in manic depression have been with Depakote (Bowden et al 2000, NICE Technology Appraisal 66). Therefore we can be confident that Depakote is an effective drug whereas the same cannot be said of other formulations of valproate. Valproate semi-sodium is a licensed treatment for mania although it currently does not have a licence in the longer term treatment of bipolar illness.

To date there have been no head-to-head trials in treating manic depression between valproate and semi-sodium valproate and so we do not know if they have the same clinical efficacy.

Valproate semi-sodium is better tolerated by the stomach than other formulations though in fact the slow-release version of sodium valproate is also a well-tolerated drug. The fact that Depakote is particularly well tolerated can be very useful in the initial stages of the treatment of mania because the dose can be escalated rapidly. Dose for dose Depakote will produce a higher blood level than other formulations of valproate.

5.34 Is carbamazepine useful in the treatment of bipolar illness?

Several anticonvulsants have been tried in the treatment of manic depression and carbamazepine has been used extensively over the last 10 years for this indication. Carbamazepine does have a licence in the UK in the treatment of manic depressive illness unresponsive to lithium. Carbamazepine is an effective antimanic treatment and is also quite sedative, particularly when it is first given, which can be an additional benefit in the early treatment of mania. The usual starting dose is 200 mg twice a day increasing up to 1 g, although sometimes higher doses are needed. Some studies showed carbamazepine to be an effective longer term preventive treatment but recent research showed that it was a less effective treatment than lithium for standard manic depressive illness (Greil et al 1997). It still has a place in the acute and long-term treatment of manic depression but should not be used in preference to lithium. However, it can be a useful alternative if lithium is neither suitable nor effective. The study by Greil et al (1997) showed that it was not as good as lithium generally, but did suggest that it may be a better treatment for schizoaffective manic depression (*see Q 1.15*)

5.35 Are there any problems in using carbamazepine?

The common side-effects of carbamazepine, particularly in the early stages of treatment, are sedation and gastrointestinal problems such as nausea. However, in the longer term it is usually a well-tolerated drug. One problem is that it induces liver enzymes: this means that carbamazepine will induce its own metabolism and sometimes the benefits of carbamazepine can wear off because of this. Commonly the enzyme induction is apparent in liver function tests so that the gamma glutamyl transferase (γGT) levels are raised. It is easy to attribute rises in γGT to being alcohol induced which is also a common complication of bipolar illness, but beware of implying this in those who are actually abstinent!

Carbamazepine also induces the metabolism of other drugs. The one that most commonly causes problems is the oral contraceptive as carbamazepine can render the oral contraceptive ineffective.

Carbamazepine also induces allergic reactions, most commonly rashes, in about 15% of those who take it. If this occurs it is usually impossible to continue with the drug and is also potentially dangerous as more serious allergic reactions can also occur including hepatitis and agranulocytosis.

5.36 Does lamotrigine have a place in the long-term treatment of manic depression?

Recent studies on lamotrigine in manic depression have been very encouraging and it seems likely that this will prove to be a more frequently used and beneficial treatment (Calabrese et al 2003). One of the main problems in treating bipolar illness is that depression is often chronic, pervasive and disabling. Lamotrigine has been shown to be an effective antidepressant in bipolar illness with only a limited propensity for switching into mania. The usual treatment dose is 200–300 mg but it can only be very slowly increased up to this level (*see Q 5.37*). This means that it is difficult to use lamotrigine in very acute depression but it can still be very useful in tackling longer term depressive symptoms. It is likely that it also has some benefit in the prevention of depression though probably not in the prevention of mania. For this reason, for those patients who have predominantly a depressive picture it is useful to consider this treatment.

5.37 Are there any problems in using lamotrigine?

 Lamotrigine has a considerable propensity for inducing allergic reactions and these are potentially life threatening. It is for this reason that a very slow introduction of the drug is needed, the usual regimen being 25 mg daily for 2 weeks, increasing to 50 mg daily for a further 2 weeks, then increase by 50 mg daily every 2 weeks up to 200 mg. Sometimes higher doses are needed and can be effective, at least up to 300 mg daily. The usual allergic reaction is a rash, though sometimes this can be of the Stevens–Johnson type which includes inflammation of the mucous membranes including the eyes. This rash can be so severe that hospitalisation and treatment with steroids is required. Very rarely fatalities have occurred. It does seem a pity that of all the anticonvulsants lamotrigine seems to be the most helpful for depression but is potentially the most dangerous.

In terms of the more predictable side-effects lamotrigine is relatively free of these and is a well-tolerated drug; however, neurological side-effects such as headache and double vision can occur.

5.38 Have any other anticonvulsants been found to be helpful in manic depression?

Because some anticonvulsants do appear to be helpful in manic depression many have been tried but none can currently be recommended for use apart from in exceptional circumstances. It is relatively common to find in manic depression (which is such a changeable disorder) that there are initial reports of benefit with new treatments but careful controlled testing does not bear out these out. Trials of gabapentin are a good example of initial reports of success which turned out not to be confirmed. Lithium also tends to come out badly in initial comparisons because the patients who are tried on new treatments are usually those who are not getting on well and so are a preselected group of lithium non-responders. Lithium has stood the test of time and it will be interesting to see which of the currently used treatments are still recommended 40 years hence!

5.39 Should anyone be taking two drugs to prevent recurrence?

If you have treated many people with manic depression you will know that there is a substantial proportion of patients who are continuing to experience recurrences or chronic symptoms despite being on one or other of the long-term preventive treatments. If this is happening then it is likely that you will be considering combining medications. Probably the most common combination is lithium with an antipsychotic, though it may be that the antipsychotic is being used as symptomatic relief for anxiety or insomnia.

There is very little information currently about whether combinations of long-term treatment are better than monotherapy. It could be that actually we should be treating bipolars with combination treatment from early on as this may lead to a better outcome, but at the moment we just do not know (see Balance Trial http://www.psychiatry.ox.ac.uk/balance/index.html).

A common tactic is to add valproate to lithium if there has been a partial response to lithium but the patient still has continuing symptoms or episodes. If this leads to a major improvement then consider withdrawing the lithium to get back to a single medication again. However, there is little scientific basis for this decision and it would be as reasonable to continue with both medications if they were both well tolerated.

5.40 Are antipsychotics useful in the long term?

A large proportion of patients who suffer from manic depression are treated with antipsychotic drugs in the long term. The reasons for this are not entirely clear, but presumably the clinicians prescribing them and the patients taking them are finding them helpful. It seems common sense that a treatment that relieves the symptoms of acute mania should also be able to prevent these symptoms returning, but there have been very few studies to test out this theory, probably because we have focused on lithium treatment.

The reasons why antipsychotics are given are probably to relieve anxiety or improve sleep, through their sedative or calming effect. Those who suffer from psychotic symptoms during mania or depression, or those with a schizoaffective disorder who experience psychotic symptoms between episodes, may find antipsychotic drugs helpful in the long term.

A few people with manic depression have very little insight and do not take regular oral medication and so, as a last resort, a depot antipsychotic is prescribed. It is likely that this does have some benefit but it would not be recommended unless other treatments were not suitable or effective.

Olanzapine is one of the few antipsychotics that has been studied in the longer term in bipolar illness (Tohen et al 2004). It has been shown to be effective in reducing manic relapse when it is continued after it has been successfully used to treat mania, and may also have some benefit in preventing depression. Some people gain weight when they are taking olanzapine and this should be tackled right from the start of treatment. It seems to cause weight gain mainly through an increase in appetite and warning patients about this and encouraging them to limit their intake of sweet foods is important. If it were not for this problem it is likely that olanzapine would be even more widely prescribed to bipolars than it already is.

Other atypical antipsychotics (e.g. quetiapine, risperidone) have proved beneficial in the acute treatment of mania and it is likely that they will also prove effective in longer term treatment.

5.41 Are there any problems with taking antipsychotics in the long term?

 Antipsychotics do cause side-effects in the long as well as the short term. The traditional antipsychotics cause anticholinergic effects including dry mouth and constipation. They also increase prolactin levels which affect menstruation, libido and bone density. Additionally, they cause movement disorders and the major problem with the long-term use of antipsychotics is the development of persistent abnormal movements – tardive dyskinesia. These are repetitive movements, usually of the face and particularly the mouth, but which can also affect other parts of the body. They are not usually distressing but are very noticeable to others so that they can be very stigmatising. The movements may reduce when the drugs are stopped but often they do not go away.

The newer (atypical) antipsychotics are much less likely to cause tardive dyskinesia; however they can still affect prolactin levels. Weight gain can be a problem with both traditional and atypical antipsychotics.

5.42 Are there special considerations for long-term treatment with lithium in the elderly?

The same long-term treatments are as appropriate for the elderly as for other adults. Complications can arise with lithium treatment because renal function slowly decreases with age. Because lithium is a salt it is not metabolised by the body but is entirely excreted by the kidney (with a small amount lost through sweat). Before starting lithium in the elderly you need to be confident that renal function is adequate, usually by undertaking a creatinine clearance test. However, the only real test is to start a small dose of lithium and check the levels while monitoring for adverse effects. The dosage of lithium is almost invariably lower, usually starting at 200 mg at night rather than 400 mg. The eventual dose is often 400–600 mg, whereas younger adults usually take 800–1200 mg daily.

Side-effects of lithium (*see* Q 5.7) are more common in the elderly, but it is as effective in this age group as for others. Similar considerations are needed for other long-term medications, where doses usually need to be lower and side-effects are often more evident.

5.43 How can compliance with treatment be improved?

Compliance is the usual name for trying to reach an agreement between doctor and patient about what treatment is appropriate. Concordance is probably a better term as it implies a real agreement rather than following medical instructions. Most relationships between doctors and patients are actually a combination of these two approaches.

The first question is: 'Are we agreed on the nature of the problem?' (Are doctor and patient agreed that the problem is manic depression, or how does the patient interpret the problems that they have run into?) If agreement cannot be reached on the problem, then it is very unlikely that there will be agreement about the treatment. No doctor wants to be in the position (that we have all been in) when doing a home visit to discover a year's worth of medication in the cupboard that the patient has been too polite to say they are not taking. The only way to avoid this is to get as good an understanding as possible as to the patient's attitudes towards their illness. It may be worth giving them more time to think about the treatment before you prescribe and ensuring that there is a long-term commitment.

If agreement cannot be reached on the specific diagnosis, can you agree on what symptoms are or were present? Sleep loss is usually a good place to start as it is easier to be objective about this compared to whether the patient is elated or irritable. Are there other symptoms that can be found that might be an agreed target for treatment (e.g. feeling restless or talking all the time)?

Even if a good level of concordance has been reached, very few people remember to take their treatment perfectly every day for months on end. It is usually better to discuss this on the assumption that it is difficult to do and to be surprised if the treatment is taken absolutely regularly. A routine is usually the best way to get round the problem of forgetting to take tablets. Can the patient link taking the treatment with some other aspect of everyday life – for example if putting the cat out each night before going to bed is part of the daily routine the patient might try leaving the pills by the back door. The more usual suggestion, however, is to leave them by the toothpaste.

Some tablet packs have the days written on them to help, but this is unusual for older drugs like lithium. Pill boxes that are filled once a week and then have a slot for each morning and evening can be a good way of helping to take the right dose each time, especially in complex regimens, and also give a good record of what has been missed.

Try to make the regimen of pill taking as easy as possible. Patients are more likely to take the pills once or twice a day rather than three or four times. For a manic patient to remember to take the medication four times a day is nearly impossible unless they have a very strict routine. It is always worth simplifying regimens as much as possible and most medications used in manic depression can be taken once a day.

Some people have trouble swallowing tablets and find capsules or liquids better. Many of the tablets (e.g. lithium) are large and taking two smaller ones may be easier. Focusing on some of these smaller issues can be particularly useful in long-term treatments as it acknowledges the difficulties involved and also gives a fairly neutral forum in which to discuss attitudes to the illness and its treatment.

5.44 What is the key to understanding the factors limiting concordance?

The fundamental problem of concordance is usually one of attitudes to treatment, rather than the practicalities. Even if doctor and patient are agreed about the diagnosis and the fact that this medicine is helpful, many bipolar patients still do not really want to take these tablets (*Case vignette 5.3*). Taking a medicine means for some people that they have failed, they don't like to have to rely on tablets to keep them stable, they're 'out of control'. It means really admitting that they have an illness, a long-term illness and they are reliant on something outside themselves, which many see as being an addict. Taking tablets can be seen as a weakness and embarrassment.

These attitudes are pretty universal and usually need discussion. Making it clear that these problems are common is a good start. Encourage patients to step outside their own situation by posing questions such as: 'What would you say to your friend who has bronchitis and has to take antibiotics, or to your brother who has diabetes and has to take insulin injections? Is that a sign of weakness or are they actually taking control of their lives rather than letting the illness dominate their lives?'

Try to spend time understanding attitudes rather than focusing on the issues that are the usual medical ones (e.g. efficacy and side-effects). Ask questions such as:

■ What treatment or help are you looking for?
■ Have you read or seen anything on television about these treatments?

- Have you ever thought that you might need to take a treatment like this?
- How ill would you need to be or how often would relapses need to occur before you would consider taking this type of treatment?
- What do you think might happen if you took this treatment?
- Do you know anything about lithium?
- Has anyone in your family (or friends) taken this treatment? How did they get on with it?
- What happened when you took this treatment before and what happened when you stopped?

It is actually pretty unusual for those who suffer a bipolar illness to take their treatment regularly right from the start and it is only after a lengthy period of time that the patient makes a decision about what treatment really is helpful and then sticks with it.

CASE VIGNETTE 5.3 BARRIER TO CONCORDANCE

Geoff clearly understood that he had manic depression and recognised that it was the same type of illness as his mother had suffered. However, he never seemed to get started on lithium, there was always some reason or excuse – he had a cold at the moment, or he hadn't managed to get the blood tests done or this wasn't a good time to start something new. Eventually he admitted that the problem was that he did not want to be like his mother. She had ended up in hospital for several years and he knew that she had taken lithium. The association in his mind was 'lithium and hospital' and that was why he was reluctant to try the treatment. Once he was able to acknowledge the problem, it was possible to make some progress with the treatment, whereas prior to that a lot of time had been spent discussing reasons which were not the real reasons.

5.45 Can other specialist staff help in the long-term management of bipolar illness?

The long-term care of manic depressives who are severely afflicted by the illness requires a range of specialist staff. At the most severe end patients can require lengthy periods of hospitalisation and also 24-hour residential care; however this is uncommon and the great majority live independently.

- *Community psychiatric nurses* can offer a wide range of interventions, the most important of which is usually their experience of how others have coped with the illness and its treatment. This advice can be invaluable, particularly in helping people to rebuild their lives after a serious breakdown. They have local knowledge and can help to reconnect people in their communities when their confidence is low. CPNs have a broad knowledge of the course of the illness, the treatments and their side-effects, which can build confidence when the patient feels they are the only one to have ever been in this situation. They can help to liaise with general practitioners to ensure that prescriptions are available and any treatment monitoring is undertaken. They usually have a broad range of psychotherapeutic skills which can help patients to understand their condition and how it relates to their life and relationships.

■ *Social workers* traditionally help with the practicalities of benefits and accommodation but also offer support to families. They are usually familiar with legal issues, both with the compulsory detention and also more unusual matters (e.g. power of attorney). If residential care is needed then they are usually responsible for organising and financing this. Many also have skills in counselling and are a good source of advice on local community services. Some social service departments employ support workers who are able to help patients with practical day-to-day tasks such as shopping and organising bills as well as other activities (e.g. going to the swimming pool).

■ *Occupational therapists* are expert at helping those recovering from mental illness to regain their skills for daily living and focus them on how they use their time and head back into the workplace.

■ *Psychologists* usually undertake specific psychotherapeutic interventions but are also able to assess intellectual and cognitive function; both to help diagnosis and to guide treatment (*see Q.5.46*).

■ *Pharmacists,* both in hospital and the community, can offer invaluable advice on medicines, how they should be taken, how they work and what interactions can occur.

Although there are a wide range of skills in a good community mental health team, the personalities of the staff are often of great importance. Having a variety of people and approaches in the team means that the full range of people who experience manic depression can be given a chance to fulfil their potential.

5.46 What psychotherapeutic approaches can help to prevent recurrence?

There are no psychotherapeutic treatments that are specific to the treatment of bipolar disorder and usually a wide range of approaches is combined to tailor the therapy to the individual patient. Two important elements in the approach of most therapists are outlined below.

IDENTIFYING THE EARLY SYMPTOMS OF RELAPSE

Many patients recognise a pattern to their illness in that certain symptoms or behaviours occur before the major relapse actually hits. If this can be identified then a plan can be made in advance as to how best to react to these symptoms (Lam et al 2003). This may be as simple as to contact a doctor or nurse to get advice or starting to take some medication. However, the essence of this approach is taking on the responsibility for managing the illness, both in terms of prevention but also at an early stage before it spirals out of control. A simple approach would be to recognise that losing sleep but lying in in the morning is usually the start of a depression. This may be the trigger for checking that the medication is being taken regularly, stopping drinking alcohol and getting advice about whether to start an antidepressant.

REVIEWING THE PAST EXPERIENCES OF TAKING AND STOPPING MEDICATION

Another technique commonly used by psychotherapists is to help patients to look at the pattern of their illness in the past. It can sometimes be very obvious to others that whenever the patient has given up lithium it has been followed by a relapse. However, this can be surprisingly difficult for patients to recognise because relapses are usually attributed to changes in personal circumstance, life's pressures or how others are behaving, and seem to be more likely explanations for mood changes. Reviewing the course of the illness can lead to a better understanding of the relationship of the illness to the variety of factors that can affect it and then lead to other solutions or at least experiments. For example this may lead to looking at taking a new medication as an experiment for 3 months. During this time the patient should keep a weekly record of mood and at the end of the period look at the record to make the judgement as to how helpful the treatment has been. This can be considerably more effective than just going on how they feel at the end of the period (*see also* Q 5.25).

 PATIENT QUESTIONS

5.47   How do I know if my lithium level is too high?

When you are taking lithium over a long period of time you will come to recognise the side-effects that typically affect you. These would usually be a mild tremor and feeling thirsty. You should be having your blood level monitored every 3 months and this should be staying at a reasonably steady level (you would not expect it to vary by more than 0.2 mmol/l above or below the regular level). If the side-effects and blood levels are steady then you should not need to worry about having toxic levels.

However, if you start to get new physical symptoms then you need to think whether these could be because the level is getting high. The first sign of high levels is stomach problems – feeling nauseous and getting diarrhoea. Stomach upsets are obviously quite common, but if you have one you need to think if this could be because the lithium level is too high. It is very easy

PQ PATIENT QUESTIONS

to get an extra blood lithium level done and if you are getting stomach problems you should do this.

If the level gets even higher you will feel generally unwell, not only being sick but getting very thirsty, more shaky and could even get unsteady on your feet and your speech start to slur as if you were drunk. These symptoms are very serious and you need to get some urgent medical advice. In the meantime, stop your lithium. You may find that the lithium level comes back as not very high – this level can only really be understood by knowing when your last dose of lithium was, and if you have not taken the lithium for a couple of days but have a 'normal' level this may well mean that you still have a lot of lithium in your body.

5.48   What happens if I stop lithium suddenly?

You have a very high chance of becoming manic if you suddenly give up lithium treatment. Probably the best way of setting off a manic spell is to take lithium for a few months then suddenly stop it. You have about a one in three chance of relapsing and it is usually into mania rather than depression.

If you are going to stop lithium, you need to do it gradually, reducing by about 200 mg every couple of weeks. However, do remember that you need to have a very good reason why you are stopping the treatment as manic depression does not go away. It may be that you have decided that you are going to change over to another treatment because the lithium does not seem to be working well or you are getting side-effects. If you are staying well on it you should not be stopping it just because it is working well!

5.49   Why should I take my lithium all at night?

Lithium does not work better if it is taken all at night. However, side-effects are usually related to how high the level is in the blood and the highest levels are in the first few hours after you take the tablets. So if you take your tablets at night it is while you are asleep that the levels are higher so you may not notice the side-effects.

The other issue is getting a blood test to check the level of lithium in the blood. The blood test needs to be taken 12 hours after the last dose. So if you take the lithium in the evening you can get a blood test in the morning. If you are taking the lithium in the morning you may find it difficult to persuade your surgery to do a blood test in the evening! Some people who find it difficult to take lithium do split the doses between morning and evening. You should then get a blood test before you take the morning dose, even if this means delaying it for a few hours.

5.50   What if I have missed a dose of lithium?

If you realise in the morning that you missed your lithium last night, then you can take the dose that morning and then take it again that night. If it is after lunch then leave it out altogether and get back to the normal regimen that night.

With other medicines the usual rule of thumb is if you take it once a day then if you miss a dose then you could take it within the next 12 hours. If it is twice a day then take it within the next 6 hours, otherwise leave it. Missing occasional doses once a week or so is unlikely to have much effect on the effectiveness of the treatment.

5.51   How long will I need to take lithium?

If you have just started lithium the first aim is to judge whether the treatment suits you. A few people are particularly sensitive to lithium and find that they just cannot get on with it even at low doses because of side-effects. You should be able to find this out in the first few weeks of treatment, though occasionally it is the long-term side-effects which mean that you cannot continue.

The next aim is to judge whether the treatment is beneficial. This usually needs to be done over 6 months to a year, so that even if you suffer a relapse in the first few months it is usually worth continuing the treatment to make a longer term judgement. You need to compare how you are over this length of time to previous periods without lithium.

If lithium does prove beneficial and acceptable then it needs to be taken long term. Manic depression never goes away and if you are doing well while on lithium there needs to be a very good reason why you are stopping it. It can prove disastrous after 10 years of being well to then have a serious relapse because you have stopped the lithium.

Some people say that it needs to be taken for life – I am not sure about this as I am not very good at predicting where life will lead us in a couple of years' time let alone in the next 50 years. My usual suggestion is that we agree that you will continue over the next 5 years but then review where things stand then: it's very difficult to make a decision for a lifetime! There may of course be other treatments that emerge in the coming years which will replace lithium or indeed provide a permanent cure – but currently lithium is still the treatment most likely to be of benefit to manic depressives.

Special circumstances and considerations

6

PQ PATIENT QUESTIONS

6.1   How can families come to terms with the illness?

There is no doubt that manic depression is a very serious, long-term illness that has a major impact on both the sufferer and the family. It puts enormous strain on close relationships and many families have been permanently ruptured by its effects. Each family finds its own way of coming to terms with the illness although there are some themes that often emerge.

Bipolar illness is usually outside of most people's experience and it is easy to mistake the signs of the illness for other problems, such as delinquency or drunkenness or just plain stupidity. It is often only much later that these behaviours can be recognised as symptoms of manic depression. Reacting to an illness is different to reacting to other problems because of the issue of responsibility. Most of us would consider our partner or adult children to be responsible for their behaviour if they are getting into arguments, losing their job or getting drunk. However, if this is because they are manic then we would think that they are less responsible for their behaviour and we would give them more leeway, tend to ignore it but focus instead on getting appropriate help and treatment. Shifting from blaming the person to blaming the illness is a major shift in attitude.

However, the next step that is often reached is how much is the person who has the bipolar illness responsible for keeping themselves well and how much falls to the family? These issues usually revolve around the patient taking medication appropriately and taking care of themselves in terms of alcohol or illicit drugs and other aspects of lifestyle.

The other tension is that the patient will generally resent everything about the way they behave being put down to their illness, so that effectively anything they say or do which is at all out of the ordinary is dismissed as a symptom of their illness.

These issues are very similar to those that occur in adolescence as parents grapple with giving their children independence to do what they want, whether it is the right thing or not!

The accusation that 'you're treating me like a child' is commonly heard. Finding the right balance at the right time is never perfectly achieved but can only be approached if both sides are able to be honest about what they think and feel. The right approach in one circumstance and in one stage of the illness may be entirely wrong in another, but finding this flexibility is very difficult. It is also easy to react with anger (on both sides) and want to walk away but this rarely works well, though occasionally is exactly right!

There are other aspects of the illness that families have to grapple with including the loss of hopes and dreams for the patient and for themselves and others in the family. Taking a realistic look at the illness and how much it will affect everyone's lives is hard as there is a lot of uncertainty, particularly in the early years. Some will tend to go down a path of denial, and this is an aspect of thinking that most families go through at some point. They may either ignore what has happened or just hope that it will not happen again. Alternatively, they may move to the other extreme and assume that normal life is now entirely over. Keeping a realistic view of the future is important, and revising it as events unfold is part of that.

6.2 What is the best way to present information to parents about the cause of bipolar disorder?

Most parents will feel guilty if their child develops a mental illness. This is partly because we all feel responsible for how our children turn out and worry about whether we have brought them up properly. In bipolar illness it is more complicated because there are strong genetic factors. Understanding the genetics of the illness can be very painful and provokes thoughts such as: 'It's all my fault, he's got this from me because I've been depressed'.

Try to put this into perspective for the parents. There are risks for all of us that our children may develop manic depression (about 1%). If a parent suffers from manic depression then there is about a 10% risk of any child having a bipolar illness. The risk of depression in the general population is about 5% but nearer 25% for the children of bipolars. Depression and bipolar illness are also very variable illnesses in their severity. These are substantial figures but on average if a manic patient had four children only one is likely to have a serious affective disorder, and there are of course many other possible illnesses for which they may be at risk (see Fig. 2.2).

6.3 Do manic depressives have cognitive or intellectual deficits?

When Kraepelin made the distinction between manic depression and schizophrenia a hundred years ago, he did it partly on the basis that there was cognitive impairment among the schizophrenic group. In fact the name he gave to the illness we now call schizophrenia was dementia praecox. This comes from the Latin, meaning a precocious or premature dementia. It is certainly true that a major disability for those who suffer from schizophrenia is an impairment of their intellectual function. The situation for bipolars is less clear.

Before the symptoms of the illness start it is commonly found, among those with schizophrenia, that their school performance has been below average. This does not seem to apply to bipolars and in fact they are likely to be somewhat above average.

It is easy to recognise the intellectual impairments of severe depression, particularly when it is accompanied by retardation where even the most basic of mental tasks (e.g. getting a few words out) is difficult. The distractibility of mania also precludes clear and effective thinking. However, when there has been a good recovery from mania and depression, is there any cognitive impairment still present? At first sight there is not, but when detailed tests of intellectual function are undertaken then abnormalities emerge. Bipolars as a group do not have the severe impairments that those with schizophrenia show but they still do not equate to normal controls. It may be that this is part of the explanation for why those with manic depression often do not seem to be doing as well at work as would be expected even though they have made a good recovery in terms of being free of manic or depressive symptoms.

There are no particular tests that bipolars are especially likely to perform poorly on that can be easily tested in the surgery and in fact the differences between bipolars and normal controls tend to be matters of degree rather than categorical differences. It is also worth remembering that even minor levels of symptoms can have a substantial effect on intellectual function and this needs to be borne in mind when considering treatment.

6.4 Are there chemical changes that occur in bipolar disorder?

The most commonly reported chemical change is an increase in cortisol in the blood during periods of depression or mania. The daily rhythm of cortisol is normally at its lowest at midnight and highest in the morning, but in severe affective states this rhythm tends to be lost with persistent high levels at night. This overproduction of cortisol is not suppressed by giving dexamethasone.

A large number of other tests, particularly of abnormalities in the amine systems of the brain (serotonin, noradrenaline (norepinephrine) and dopamine), have been looked at in both bipolar illness and more commonly in depression which suggest that there may be underlying changes in these systems. However, this work is very difficult to do because of the urgency of treating patients in severe affective states and the effects of medications on these systems. It is for these reasons that a coherent and consistent account of brain chemical abnormalities has yet to emerge. It is common to hear that manic depression is caused by a chemical imbalance in the brain but rare to hear exactly what this imbalance is. We tend to assume that because a lot of the drugs we use affect the amine systems that manic depression is a problem in these systems and that the drugs correct this. Lithium is a very basic challenge to this idea, and we still do not know with any certainty how this treatment works.

6.5 Do complementary treatments have a place?

Where the line between mainstream and complementary treatment is drawn is uncertain. We are still not sure what forms of 'talking' therapies are effective (*see Qs 3.20 and 5.46*) and many people find less specialist forms of talking useful, from non-directive counselling to assertiveness training and anger management.

■ *Alternative medicines*: There are really no good data to guide advice on alternative drugs or foods in bipolar illness, but it is inevitable that some patients are taking them as the market is huge. Often the treatments that are used in depression such as St John's wort are tried in manic depression. St John's wort has been shown to be of benefit in mild depression and so it seems likely that it would also help bipolar depression, but like other antidepressants it may also have the propensity to destabilise bipolar disorder (*see Table 3.2*). There are also concerns that there can be interactions with other drugs, and so if St John's wort is being taken it should probably not be mixed with mainstream drugs. It is difficult to give advice on other herbs apart from exercising caution.

■ *Vitamins and minerals*: Vitamins and other mineral supplements are also popular but should not be seen as a substitute for a healthy diet. However, some bipolar patients with a severe and chronic illness can become malnourished and taking multivitamins would seem sensible. Those who also have complicating alcohol problems may well benefit from B vitamins.

■ *Omega 3 fatty acids*: Omega 3 fatty acids, usually found in fish oil, are popular for both rheumatological and psychiatric disorders and there have been some encouraging trials in manic depression (Stoll et al 1999). The doses recommended in the clinical trials have been high and most readily available preparations will not provide these high levels. These may well become mainstream treatments in the future.

■ *Relaxation therapy*: Being able to relax is a great advantage to anyone who has problems with anxiety which includes most bipolars. Many complementary therapies, including aromatherapy, yoga, tai chi and massage have a strong relaxation element to them which can make them very helpful.

■ *Homeopathy*: Some alternative practitioners recommend that all medicines are stopped but this can be very counterproductive. There does not appear to be any evidence that homeopathy is effective in bipolar disorder.

6.6 How does the stigmatisation of mental illness affect manic depressives?

Stigma means a mark of social disgrace. It is a form of prejudice that means making negative assumptions about people. It has a major impact on those who experience mental illness including those with manic depression. The common views are that they have brought the illness on themselves and that they are likely to be dangerous and violent.

There are also some rather paradoxical ideas – for example thinking that depression is a sign of weakness and that people should just 'pull themselves together' while at the same time thinking that nothing can be done to improve mental illnesses and therefore it will permanent. These views are so common and pervasive that many people with the illness will also share those ideas and so not think that it is worth bothering trying to get some help or treatment (*see also Q 5.44*).

The other view that people who have bipolar illness commonly hear is – 'You don't seem like the type of person to suffer from depression' – which chimes with the idea that only certain people can experience mental illness (*see Q 1.18*).

The practical effect of stigma is that people are not given a chance to show what they can or cannot do – it's just assumed that they are incapable. It is also very corrosive to someone's self-esteem to be dismissed on the basis of assumptions about their illness.

Obviously manic depression does have a disabling effect on everyone that experiences it and it can lead to extreme, bizarre and unpredictable behaviour. This is part of the illness and needs to be faced and tackled head on, although stigma does exaggerate the disability.

Education about the illness and getting to know people who suffer from manic depression seem to be the only ways to reduce stigma. Learning about the reality of bipolar disorder and the ordinariness of those who experience it can change attitudes. One of the most powerful ways that stigma can be tackled is by prominent people letting it be known that they suffer from manic depression. In the United States, Ted Turner, who founded CNN (the news network), made it public that he suffered from the illness. In the UK, Spike Milligan was not only open about his illness (*Case vignette 6.1*) but also became patron of the Manic Depression Fellowship.

CASE VIGNETTE 6.1 TACKLING STIGMA

Spike Milligan is one of the few people in the UK to have been open about his manic depression. If you are familiar with his comedy you might think that his main problem was mania but in fact like most bipolars it was depression that really dogged him. At least some of his writing was driven by his manic or hypomanic symptoms but he said that his comic genius was not worth the manic depression agony.

Spike had a family history of depression in his mother who was depressed after his birth. He had a difficult childhood with his mother's problems and his father being away in the army. He spent his early years in India and found it a shock to return to a cold and harsh pre-war England.

He joined the army in World War II and fought for 4 years in North Africa and Italy before being wounded in a mortar attack. Following this he was 'weepy, frightened, lethargic and ill'. He was treated with tranquillisers and after a week was sent back – 'Up to the guns and as soon as I heard them go I started to stammer'. He was withdrawn from frontline service.

As a young man he was prone to mood swings, 'fast and joking' at times but 'low and lacking drive' at others.

He developed his career after the War, particularly as the writer of *The Goon Show* in the 1950s. He seemed to do this in a frenzy of activity with at times very little sleep in an intense and highly productive 6 years. Towards the end of this time he was probably manic but he collapsed into depression and was admitted to hospital.

Over the following years he had several admissions to hospital and his depressions were long and debilitating. His illness was severe enough to require treatment with ECT. Mania was not a prominent part of his illness but he seems to have used his manic energy productively.

He died in 2002, and the epitaph he chose for his gravestone reads: 'I told you I was ill'.

His manic humour is revealed in the way that he played with words and ideas – for example 'This is Minnie Bannister, the world-famous poker player – give her a good poker and she'll play any tune you like.'

6.7 Should patients be given drug holidays?

Several people have suggested that taking a break from medication might be a good strategy as it could minimise any long-term ill effects of the treatment and stop the beneficial effect wearing off. This may have some intuitive appeal as an idea but is in practice very likely to lead to more relapses and a worse outcome (*see Case vignette 5.2*) and following this line should be strongly discouraged. In particular nobody should stop lithium suddenly as there is a very high chance of relapse into mania (*see Q 5.27*).

There are particular problems with treating patients with antipsychotics in the long term in that there is a substantial risk of tardive dyskinesia (abnormal involuntary movements which are usually permanent). However, if this type of treatment is needed in the long term then, rather than giving drug holidays, consideration should be given to using the newer atypical antipsychotics which have a lower risk of this disorder developing (*see Q 5.41*).

6.8 What is the future direction for treatments for manic depression?

We have the same hopes for the treatment of manic depression that we do for most other illnesses. Molecular biology offers the possibility of a more profound understanding of the condition and the potential to create more specific treatments.

One line that may prove fruitful in the near future is choosing treatments according to genotype. Not all treatments are as effective in one person as in another and if we can discover the genetic associations of this, then we may be able to give more specific advice about what medications are likely to be useful for a specific individual.

The sad truth is that we are not using the treatments that we have at the moment to best effect. This is most apparent in the research that has looked at suicide in bipolar patients (Isometsa et al 1994, Schou 1998). Most bipolars who kill themselves have either not been prescribed appropriate long-term treatment or have not been taking it.

We need to improve our general skills as doctors so that we are better at recognising the condition, teaching our patients to understand their illness and finding the best ways of minimising their disability. Research on psychotherapeutic approaches may also tell us what specific areas we should be focusing on and techniques we should be using.

6.9   What is self-management?

Everyone with a serious chronic illness needs to find a way to understand and manage that illness so that the disabling effect on their life is minimised.

The term 'self-management' has been used by the Manic Depression Fellowship (MDF, *see Appendix 1*) for this process of gaining more control over the condition. The MDF is a national self-help organisation in the UK. They promote this process of taking more responsibility for one's own condition through literature, self-help groups and a national training course.

There are a number of elements in self-management:

1. The first is the recognition of what can set off another episode of illness and what are the early signs of relapse. This needs to be not only a general understanding of the illness but also a specific knowledge of how the illness affects the individual.
2. If the early indications are recognised then a plan should be implemented to:
    — deal with the symptoms
    — minimise the problems that are likely to arise
    — find the people that can help
    — make the appropriate changes in medication to either abort the episode or reduce its impact.
3. People are also encouraged to minimise the possibility of relapse through promoting lifestyle changes and taking appropriate medication. They are encouraged to develop a personalised action plan to put what they learn about themselves and their illness into effect.

Being an informed and insightful patient is undoubtedly one of the best routes to long-term mental stability for those with bipolar illness.

6.10   What is the interaction between the medications used in treating bipolar illness and alcohol?

Many of the drugs used to treat bipolar disorder have sedative effects; this is true not only of the antipsychotics and benzodiazepines but also the anticonvulsants, particularly carbamazepine. Alcohol tends to enhance these sedative effects and can also exaggerate other CNS side-effects, such as ataxia. There is no direct interaction with lithium unless alcohol is drunk to the level of causing dehydration which can raise lithium levels.

Some antidepressants, particularly trazodone and the sedative tricyclics such as amitriptyline and dosulepin (dothiepin), are also likely to enhance drowsiness when taken with alcohol. SSRIs are generally less sedative and the interaction is likely to be less.

Doctors often feel in a dilemma when discussing alcohol use with people who suffer from manic depression. Patients need to have information about interactions but doctors do not want to be seen to encourage alcohol as so many patients have problems with excessive drinking. Most longer term medications do not prevent drinking modest amounts of alcohol. There is an element of trial and error because individuals vary in their tolerance of alcohol and medicines. Patients will usually find that they can tolerate a moderate amount of alcohol in combination with their medication.

Heavy restrictions on alcohol are difficult to comply with as so much social life revolves around drinking alcohol and most of us like to drink. If patients feel doctors have unrealistic views about alcohol then they probably will not be frank about their alcohol use.

On the other hand, it is easy to collude with excessive drinking and if you can help someone tackle a common problem early then you are doing them a real favour. Discussions that help them to explore non-alcohol-related avenues of social contact, or even experimenting with not drinking, can be useful lines to follow. But one needs to stay realistic as alcohol use is so pervasive in our culture that even when people do get involved with other activities (e.g. playing squash), they find that they are expected to go and have a drink afterwards!

6.11 What is the effect of bipolar illness on work?

Those who are acutely ill with depression or mania will usually be too disabled to work, either because their concentration and attention are not sufficient or their judgement is poor. In the longer run it is disappointing to see that only about a quarter of manic depressives seem to be able to maintain work at a level at which their qualifications and experience would suggest they are capable. The reasons for this include the direct effects of the illness on the ability to work and the attitude of others. The disruptions that acute episodes of illness can cause are the most obvious effect. Manic episodes that involve embarrassing and irresponsible behaviour can prove very disruptive to working relationships that thrive on trust. Even after recovery from an acute episode low level depressive symptoms are common and this can impact on the motivation and innovation that productive work requires. Some people have mild cognitive deficits which prevent them performing at the level that would be expected, even if they have apparently made a good recovery from their mood symptoms. Many patients feel that the medications they are taking are affecting their cognitive ability or their enthusiasm or creativity. These are aspects of medication that are not well described or investigated and it is very difficult to disentangle effects of medications from long-term symptoms.

The attitude of employers makes an enormous difference; those that are sympathetic, often because they have had emotional problems themselves, can be enormously helpful in promoting achievement at work. More commonly employers can prove very negative and obstructive and really prevent people who have made a good recovery from returning to work. Those who will allow patients to test out their abilities by coming back to work on a gradual basis, both in terms of responsibility and time, usually get the best out of those with bipolar illness. However, in jobs that require a high degree of responsibility and independence, including medicine, it is often difficult to put into place the required supervision and monitoring that would enable people to practise effectively and safely.

It is easy for people with bipolar illness to take very low key jobs in an attempt to avoid stress and because their self-esteem is poor. Unfortunately boring jobs can prove just as stressful as more responsible ones. Try to encourage people to find a way of making a reasonable assessment of their abilities, perhaps by asking a colleague who knows them well. Those with bipolar illness should aim to work to the best of their abilities rather than assume that they have to go for a job with lower expectations.

6.12 What are the rules on driving?

Doctors need to make an assessment of the fitness of a patient to drive at that particular time and give consideration to the longer term. Those who are acutely ill with mania or depression should not drive because of judgement and concentration problems and they need to be told this. This assessment can be very obvious when people are severely ill but is much harder to judge at milder levels of illness. Doctors need to consider not only the level of illness at the time the patient is seen, but also their recent behaviour. The account of others such as family and their view of the risk can be very informative. Also consider whether the illness is likely to get worse as judged by the severity of previous episodes and, if the illness is settling, that sufficient time is allowed to be confident that there will not be a relapse.

Driving can be such an important part of life, particularly for those who live in more rural areas where public transport is limited, that doctors are loath to prevent driving. However, this needs to be balanced by the risks that driving entails. Patients are far more likely to injure themselves or someone else in the course of their driving than they are because of direct violence.

The author's usual rule is to consider people fit, even if they have had a severe episode, if they have made a good recovery, which has been sustained for 3 months, and as long as the medication they are taking is not interfering with their ability to drive. This judgement is usually made on the basis of observations and the report of the patient, and again making use of a relative if this is possible.

All patients with manic depression should be encouraged to contact the licensing authorities. In the UK the way to do this is set out on the driving licence documents. Patients should give the authorities the names of doctors who can provide evidence about their fitness to drive. Tell patients that this is a legal requirement and that their licence is not valid, and neither is their insurance, if they have not informed the authorities of any serious illness which includes manic depression. This has the advantage of not only being true but putting some independent decision making into the process rather than you being the sole arbiter.

Doctors also have to make judgements along with patients on the effects of medication and most of the medications used in bipolar illness can impair attention and concentration and so driving ability. This is often particularly true when the treatment is started. Particular care should be taken about benzodiazepines which are commonly found in the blood of those involved in car accidents. Many patients think that taking the medicine is what is stopping them driving whereas it is usually the opposite: it is regular compliance with treatment that is necessary for them to be fit to drive regularly again.

6.13 Are manic depressives more creative than other people?

Both mania and depression do lead to people thinking about themselves and their situation in different ways from those of us who have never experienced these extremes of mood. This insight can certainly be used creatively but the usual barrier to this is the difficulty in concentration and motivation which is so much a part of acute manic depressive illnesses. The increased energy of hypomania can improve productivity and the combination of fast thinking and distractibility can lead to innovations in thinking and ideas. Several famous poets, novelists and artists have suffered extremes of mood, particularly depression, which some think is linked to their creativity (Jamison 1994). Schubert is the composer who is often cited as a classic example of a manic depressive whose levels of productivity and creativity varied dramatically from year to year according to his mood state.

On the other hand, the sad truth is that most people who suffer from manic depression have their creativity badly stifled by the illness so that productive work and family life are curtailed because of the disruption of the illness. Creative people come in all different shapes, sizes and temperaments and it is doubtful that there is anything inherent in manic depression that makes people more creative than others. There is some evidence suggesting that those who are close relatives of someone with manic depression tend to be more successful in their careers than the average. However, it is always difficult to interpret these studies because they can be very selective in which families are investigated.

> *Patient comment*: 'I have all the great ideas but I can't put them into practice.'

6.14 What are the issues around manic depression and contraception?

The most important issue is to ensure that women who are taking treatments for their bipolar illness are also taking adequate contraceptive measures. All these drugs are potentially teratogenic and some – particularly lithium, valproate and carbamazepine – have very substantial risks to the foetus (*see Q. 5.22*).

It is easy to forget about contraception when a woman has been seriously ill and the focus is on the treatment of her mental illness, which can prove very complex. It is worth remembering that increased libido and sexual disinhibition are common symptoms of mania and hypomania. The other related risk is of sexually transmitted diseases which is relevant for males as well as females.

Often when female patients are manic they will not remember to take oral contraceptive pills and consideration of other modes of delivery (e.g. long-acting injection or intrauterine device) may be needed.

There is a particular concern with carbamazepine which is a potent inducer of liver enzymes. This enzyme induction can reduce levels of the hormones in the oral contraceptive and so render it ineffective. Higher dose pills are therefore likely to be needed when taken in combination with carbamazepine.

6.15 What advice should be given to a woman with manic depression who wants to have a baby?

There are two main aspects to this advice:

■ the risk of illness during pregnancy and after childbirth
■ the potential effects of medication on the growing foetus.

Women remain at risk of suffering acute episodes of mania or depression during pregnancy though the risk may be slightly reduced when compared to other times. However, the reduction in risk is small and it should not be assumed that pregnancy is protective against manic depression. On the other hand, the risk of relapse (particularly of manic relapse after childbirth) is very high, perhaps eight times the risk of any other month. Most women with manic depressive illness will need to take some preventive medication during pregnancy. Only those who have infrequent episodes are likely to get through pregnancy without a relapse and without medication.

There is always a concern about taking any medication during pregnancy because of the risks to the foetus. However, there are very particular concerns of foetal abnormality with lithium and anticonvulsants including valproate and carbamazepine. These risks need to be carefully explained to potential mothers, and this should be recorded in the notes as it is a common source of legal problems for doctors.

Lithium is well known to be teratogenic, but it is difficult to get firm figures for this risk. It is likely that the early estimates of risk were inflated because of how the data were gathered. However, the mother should be aware that taking lithium triples the risk of abnormality in the foetus and that there is about a 10% risk of a serious physical problem.

Valproate and carbamazepine are associated with neural tube defects in about 1% of births. Valproate is slightly more dangerous than carbamazepine. It may be that taking folate can mitigate this risk and this is advised prior to and during pregnancy. Antidepressants and antipsychotic drugs, particularly the older ones, are of less risk to the foetus, though there are now reassuring data that fluoxetine is also a lower risk treatment (*see* www.ncl.ac.uk/pharmsc/entis.htm).

The risks to the foetus from the medication do need to be balanced against the risks to the foetus and the mother if she relapses. Acute mania or depression will almost always require medication, often at higher doses and with more than one medication. Thus the aim of preventing exposure of the foetus to medication can actually lead to higher levels of treatment than if the preventive medication had been continued. This is coupled with the effect on the physical health of the mother through poor self-care during an acute episode.

The discussions with a woman who wishes to get pregnant (or who presents already pregnant) are never easy and only a mother can weigh up the risks of taking or not taking medication.

The safest tactic is to try to reduce and stop the medication prior to pregnancy. This is not always easy and the situation often arises of trying to take a woman slowly off preventive medication in order for her to become pregnant only to find that she relapses each time and has to restart treatment.

6.16 What special measures need to be taken when a pregnant woman is continuing to take medication?

If the mother has decided to continue preventive treatment during pregnancy despite the risks to the foetus because the chance of relapse without treatment is high, then you need to ensure that the obstetric team is aware of the medication and the reason for it. It is likely that the degree of monitoring of the foetus will be increased to detect any defects at an early stage.

In the case of valproate and carbamazepine you must ensure that the woman is taking folate before becoming pregnant, as this can reduce the incidence of neural tube defects.

Monitoring of mental state and medication needs to continue but at a higher level of vigilance. The levels of lithium can vary with pregnancy and often decrease with changes in body fluid and renal excretion. This may mean that a higher dose needs to be given to preserve the prophylactic effect. This should be borne in mind after delivery as the levels can rise as these effects reverse.

You need to ensure that you record your discussion in your records as this is an area that commonly leads to litigation.

6.17 What is the risk of relapse after childbirth?

The risk of relapse after childbirth is the highest in a woman's life; at least a third of women with manic depression will relapse at this time (Freeman et al 2002). When making plans for the period after childbirth the assumption should be that the relapse will occur and there needs to be either very close monitoring or early initiation of preventive treatment. This needs to be judged according to the past history but puerperal illness can start very suddenly and the potential consequences to the mother and child are enormous. There are tragedies each year of new mothers dying through suicide or the mother seriously harming the child and rarely even killing them in a psychotic state. Although these incidents are rare they should be considered preventable.

Spouses are usually the main source of support and monitoring along with others including health visitors. They all need to be aware of the potential for severe relapse and a plan to take early action is the best insurance.

6.18 What is puerperal psychosis?

The puerperium is defined as the first 3 months after childbirth. This is the time in a woman's life when she is most likely to suffer a relapse of manic depression. Mania is more common than depression though both occur as do mixed states. For about a third of all women who suffer from manic depression, the puerperium is the time when they first experience a serious episode of mania or depression.

A puerperal illness can be somewhat unusual in that the symptoms vary markedly throughout a single day. For example, when seeing a mother at one time in the day she can appear fairly rational and her symptoms not be prominent, but when seeing her a few hours later she can be clearly psychotic and disturbed (*Case vignette 6.2*). The other common feature of a puerperal psychosis is confusion so that mothers can have difficulty saying what day or what time it is, have trouble recognising people or places and getting lost in familiar surroundings.

The recognition and treatment of puerperal psychosis is vital for the health of both mother and baby and it is for this reason that there are specific mother-and-baby psychiatric beds in many (but unfortunately as yet not all) parts of the country. Successful treatment of a newly delivered psychotic mother can also prove exceptionally rewarding as she will usually make a good recovery.

The treatment of puerperal psychosis is essentially the same as treatment of mania or depression at other times, antipsychotics usually being the basis of medication treatment because manic and psychotic symptoms are so common. Some psychiatrists say that electroconvulsive therapy is particularly indicated at this time as it is a treatment of rapid onset and effectiveness, enabling the mother to recover as quickly as possible.

CASE VIGNETTE 6.2 RECOGNISING PUERPERAL PSYCHOSIS

Alice delivered her second child 3 weeks ago. She had some problems with depression after the first baby but got by without any treatment. The only known family history is of an aunt who ended up in an asylum but this was not really talked about in the family.

She has not slept well since the baby was born. The baby has actually been pretty good and usually only wakes once during the night, but after she has fed him she cannot get back to sleep because her mind is so active, worrying whether something will happen to him. She has lost her confidence as a mother and her husband is having to help. This is very unlike her as she is usually very competent both at home and in her work as a nurse.

The midwife had called but at that visit Alice had seemed fine and although the midwife was concerned, she felt that Alice was at last getting on top of her problems. However, later that evening she was spraying her breast milk at her 3-year-old daughter, which she later denied, saying it was ridiculous to think that she would do such a thing.

Alice has now not slept for three nights and 'doesn't seem to know what's going on'. She phoned her mother to come and help but called her a 'fucking bitch' when she arrived. The midwife returned to find that Charlotte was half naked in the kitchen saying that someone had been banging on the back door demanding sex.

6.19 Can women breast feed if they are taking medications for bipolar disorder?

If the mother is taking lithium then it is likely that the baby will have substantial lithium blood levels and may suffer toxicity, so breast feeding should be strongly discouraged (*see Q. 5.24*). The advice on valproate and carbamazepine is less clear and probably only small amounts get into the baby, though this can still cause problems (e.g. developing a drug-related rash).

Everyone advises caution with antidepressants and antipsychotics, especially newer drugs where we have few data. On balance most doctors would advise women to bottle rather than breast feed if they are taking these medications. However, this is an area that many women feel strongly about and in every case a thorough discussion needs to take place.

6.20 What is different about treating adolescents with bipolar disorder?

Diagnosis can be a difficult issue in this age group. There are a lot of other changes going on for teenagers and irritability is commonly seen. There is a natural reluctance to give a mental illness diagnosis and pursue a line of medication use unless you are sure that this is correct. Adolescents have the same symptoms as adults although adolescents may be more likely to have psychotic ideas and mixed affective states (*see Q 1.11*).

Treating adolescents with almost any medical condition can be stormy. This is often related to feeling angry and resentful at having a serious illness when their peers are all fit and healthy. Teenagers are usually keen to show their independence, make their own decisions and take care of themselves. Giving advice to them about treatment and lifestyle can often lead to resistance! It is usually difficult for them to fully recognise the nature of their illness and how little control they can have over their emotional state. People who suffer from bipolar illness need to take much better care of themselves than their peers do, which can be another source of resentment. Sticking to treatment regimens is difficult for everyone but teenagers can find it particularly arduous.

Illicit drug use is common among those in their teens and twenties and more common among those who have a mental illness. This can not only affect the course of the illness but also lead to other health and sometimes legal problems (*Case vignette 6.3*).

On the other hand, adolescents can also prove very robust and often manage to make up for lost time when they do recover. There is no reason to think that treatments that are effective for adults should not be used for adolescents, but as in the rest of medicine there are few treatment studies in this age group to guide the choice of drugs.

CASE VIGNETTE 6.3 DRUG USE AND NON-COMPLIANCE CAN BE SERIOUS COMPLICATIONS FOR ADOLESCENTS

Emelia had some problems at school when she was making and selling CDs to her friends. She had taken their money on the promise of making the CDs but found that she could not get them all made on time and her equipment broke down. The other students reported her to the school, who had contacted her parents and also the police. Her parents thought she had not been right but a psychiatric assessment indicated that this was unlikely to be related to any mental illness.

Three years later she presented in an emergency, having been ejected from a hotel where she had thrown a television through a third storey window. She had got fed up with all the programmes going on about her when it was none of their business. She was admitted to hospital and found to be irritable, sleepless and paranoid. She admitted smoking cannabis regularly and occasionally taking cocaine. Her symptoms settled over 4 weeks with antipsychotic treatment.

Over the next 3 years she had three further admissions and on each occasion she was both elated and irritable, as well as being overactive, aggressive and paranoid. Though she made a good recovery at each admission and managed to get back to college (they were particularly indulgent of her illness as she had a considerable artistic talent) she continued to smoke cannabis regularly and did not take any medication unless strongly encouraged by her parents. She also continued to have some unusual ideas about the way that television programmes would mention her name in obscure ways and had made a compilation video tape of these, which no-one else found very convincing (*see also Q 1.15*).

6.21 How should anxiety be treated in someone with a bipolar illness?

Anxiety is a common problem for those suffering from manic depression and at least a quarter of manic depressives report this. The first line of assessment and treatment is to look at whether there are prominent symptoms of depression. Anxiety is a common part of depression and if there is a full depressive syndrome then treatment would proceed as usual for bipolar depression.

However, others experience marked anxiety but do not have prominent depressive symptoms and the anxiety needs to be treated in its own right. A first step is to look at lifestyle factors, particularly the use of alcohol and caffeine. On the medication front antidepressants are usually the treatments of choice for anxiety disorders but the risk of precipitating mania should always be borne in mind (*see Q 3.15*). Benzodiazepines are effective anxiolytics in the short term but the risks of tolerance and dependence mean that these treatments should be used for a few weeks at the most.

Psychological approaches to managing anxiety can be effective though they are probably less so in those with manic depression than in those with uncomplicated anxiety disorders. However, everyone suffering from an anxiety disorder should be familiar with a relaxation technique that they find effective and the basics of anxiety management which can be found in a self-help book (*see Further reading* and Turner 2004).

6.22 Do people with manic depression have evidence of brain damage?

Studies that have compared patients with psychotic illnesses including schizophrenia and manic depression with normal controls have consistently shown that there is a statistical increase in the amount of fluid in the ventricles of the brain and surrounding it. This indicates that there is, on average, some loss of brain matter in those with psychosis compared with controls. This is more markedly so in those suffering from schizophrenia than with manic depression.

The differences between bipolars and normal controls are statistical rather than categorical; in other words it is not possible to tell from any brain scan whether the person is in the bipolar or the control group. There is often a difficulty in finding appropriate controls for comparison and some studies have tended to compare patients to 'super normal' people who have been heavily screened to exclude any possible factor that might affect the brain, rather than just the guy who lives next door!

Magnetic resonance imaging (MRI) studies have also tended to show an increase in abnormalities in the brain. These show up as intense white spots on the scans. These hyperintensities occur in the white matter of the brain and are often present even in the early stages of bipolar illness in those who have made a good recovery from the acute episode. We do not know what these abnormalities mean or why they occur. It has been thought that these may relate to vascular changes in the brain, though they can be present in those bipolars who do not appear to be particularly liable to vascular disease. It would be easy to assume that these lesions would be related to cognitive impairment but so far this has not been shown to be the case (Monkul et al 2003).

It is not apparent that there is a particular area of the brain which is abnormal that might be considered as the 'seat' of manic depression.

Many people with manic depression and their families ask that their brain be scanned to see if there is any abnormality. Many psychiatrists will perform brain scans particularly of new patients with manic depression to make sure that there is no organic abnormality but the pick-up of identifiable lesions is low and that of remediable lesions is even lower.

6.23 What is the treatment for rapid cycling?

Taking antidepressants is strongly associated with rapid cycling (*Fig. 6.1*) and the best line of treatment is to stop the antidepressant. There is also a connection associated with thyroid dysfunction and this should be checked as well.

It is very unusual for a patient to start the illness in a rapid cycling phase, so those who go into rapid cycling will usually have already been treated with lithium. If not, then lithium should be considered. Valproate is generally thought to be a more effective treatment than lithium for rapid cycling, though this may be partly a selection bias in the studies in that the rapid cyclers are already lithium non-responders. It may require a combination of the two mood stabilisers to bring about a resolution. Carbamazepine is the other option in trying to find a long-term treatment for the illness.

The good news about rapid cycling is that it is not a state that manic depressives stay in long term and that even if the treatment doesn't change it, rapid cycling does seem to resolve though it may transform into chronic depression. Rapid cycling is comparatively rare: at any one time less than 5% of manic depressives will be in a rapid cycling phase. It also seems to be associated with bipolar II illness so that patients are moving between depression and hypomanic states rather than the more severe manic states.

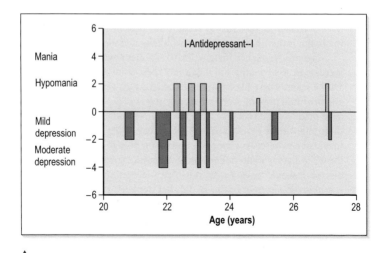

▲

Fig. 6.1 Illustration of the course of rapid cycling, in this case induced by antidepressants.

6.24 How common are substance misuse problems among manic depressives?

Rates of all commonly misused drugs are at least double (and several studies suggest at least four times higher) among bipolars compared to the general population. This is as true for nicotine addiction through cigarette smoking as it is for alcohol and illicit drugs. As with the general population, men are more likely than women to run into these problems.

It is likely that the illness leads to increased use of psychoactive drugs rather than the drugs causing the illness, as there is a rise in the rate of drug misuse following the onset of the illness. However, there is also an effect of drugs and alcohol on the course of the illness, exacerbating both mania and depression.

Those who have problems with alcohol or drugs are less likely to be compliant with their treatment and are at higher risk of suicide. It is such a common problem in this group of patients and the consequences are so serious that it needs to be routinely enquired about in all bipolars. However, it is also not uncommon to see reductions in alcohol use in the depressive phase of bipolar disorder, either as part of a general withdrawal from social situations or sometimes because patients recognise that alcohol makes them feel worse and more 'out of control'.

6.25 How should alcohol problems in bipolars be treated?

The principles of treatment for alcohol misuse and dependence are the same as for anyone else. The particular issue for most manic depressives is that they experience a predominance of dysphoric mood and so want to relieve or escape from this in any way that they can; alcohol offers a considerably more rapid relief than any of the medications we offer. However, chronic heavy alcohol use leads to more depression and withdrawal symptoms usually include anxiety. These depressive and anxiety symptoms tend to be attributed to the manic depression and alcohol seen as the only route to release. At the other end of the mood spectrum, mania causes disinhibition and drunkenness is a common consequence of this. Alcohol can then lead to escalating disruptive or aggressive behaviour.

STAGES OF MANAGEMENT

The first stage of management is recognition; it is easy to overlook alcohol problems when you are focused on serious mood disturbance but this should be borne in mind with all bipolars because excessive drinking is so common.

Though some dependent drinkers will deny problems it is not usually difficult to recognise those with dependent alcohol problems who have the features of craving alcohol, tolerance to its effects and withdrawal symptoms when they don't drink. Management of dependence will usually need to include using benzodiazepines (e.g. diazepam and chlordiazepoxide) when they stop drinking to minimise withdrawal symptoms.

Looking for lower levels of problem drinking needs to be a routine enquiry in the ongoing care of someone with manic depression. Try to find out specifically what they are drinking and how often:

- Do they drink every day?
- What is the longest they have gone without a drink?
- Why do they drink – is it to relieve anxiety or promote sleep or just 'an escape'?
- Have they considered drinking less?
- What have they tried to do already?

TREATMENT

Discuss the fact that it is a common problem for bipolars and that you want to make sure that their alcohol intake doesn't slowly creep up as a preventive strategy. Many people minimise the problems and it is only by coming back to the subject over the longer term will you be able to get them to accept that a change is needed.

The specific issues related to manic depression also need consideration. Drinking alcohol to excess is a common feature of the acute phase of both mania and depression. It may be that alcohol use between episodes is at a reasonable level. In that case the priority in treatment will be to manage the acute symptoms and if the patient can be persuaded to do this then the alcohol excess will come back under control as they recover.

More commonly the alcohol misuse will be an important factor in preventing recovery from the depression, and so reducing alcohol use is the priority. This involves two main approaches:

- Encourage a trial of abstinence to see how this affects the mood. This only requires patients to commit to a short-term change and there is a fair chance that, contrary to their expectations, their mood actually improves and they gain more stability. This will hopefully show that the alcohol is actually worsening their mood in the longer term, even though they find it gives relief in the hours after they take it. Alternatively, the medication may prove more effective when the effect of alcohol is removed. It is often also said that alcohol prevents antidepressants working properly. It is certainly true that giving up alcohol in itself has a beneficial effect on depression.

■ Maximise the benefits that can be obtained from the treatments for the bipolar illness, particularly the longer term preventive treatments, but commonly also treating low grade depressive symptoms. This is an appealing strategy, especially if it means that the patient does not need to reduce their drinking; however it is rarely successful unless attempts to reduce the drinking are also made.

Finally, be aware that alcoholism accompanying bipolar illness puts the patient at particularly high risk for suicide.

6.26 How should drug misuse in a bipolar patient be managed?

The same principles apply to drug misuse as to alcohol misuse: give the appropriate treatments and help that would be offered for the individual problems. In practice, however, this is usually difficult, the main reason being that drug misuse and manic depression make each other worse.

Substance misuse worsens the prognosis of bipolar illness because episodes of illness and psychotic symptoms can be induced by the pharmacological effect of the drug. It is also much less likely that the patient will take the medicines regularly if they are frequently intoxicated.

STAGES OF MANAGEMENT

The first stage of management is recognition; it is easy to overlook these problems when you are focused on serious mood disturbance, particularly mania. The symptoms of mania and of stimulant use are often indistinguishable and it is possible to feel confident of the diagnosis but not be sufficiently aware of the drug misuse. This should be borne in mind because drug misuse is common, particularly in young people. Some patients who have not used drugs for several years revert to them when they become manic but deny it, minimise it or forget to mention it. They may still be rather ashamed of using drugs even when they are manic and be evasive of testing. It is relatively easy nowadays to test urine for drugs in the surgery with dipsticks. Many doctors find it difficult to ask patients to give a urine sample. One approach is: 'I know that you'd previously had a problem with drugs when you were ill before/earlier in this spell, and it would be reassuring for me to know that they are entirely out of your system.' However, it is a common experience never to reach an entirely frank exchange about drug use.

Next, assess the severity of the substance misuse:

■ What are they taking, how often and in what circumstances?
■ Are they addicted – is there craving, tolerance and withdrawal symptoms?

■ Was this a problem that was apparent before the manic depression developed or is it closely related to dysphoric or elevated mood states?

TREATMENT

The initial line of treatment is to find out how serious a problem the patient perceives it to be and have a discussion about the consequences that are already apparent and what may be ahead. Many bipolars will recognise that others see drug misuse as a problem but feel they cannot tackle it because it is one of the few ways they have of gaining relief. This can be particularly true of cannabis use, which is rarely perceived as deleterious. Unless you can be agreed on the nature of the problem it is very difficult to make further progress and treatment suggestions will tend to fall on deaf ears. If this is the stage patients are at, you will need to continue to focus on the problems and consequences along with looking at any efforts they have made to tackle it. Ask about periods when they have not used drugs: – how did they get on, what other ways did they use to deal with unpleasant emotions?

If there is a clear addiction to opiates then substitution and detoxification are likely to be required if they are to stop using the drug. Opiate withdrawal is usually managed by specialists, either psychiatrists or specialist general practitioners, because of both the clinical and the legal issues involved. Stimulant and cannabis withdrawal are not usually treated with medication.

Managing the interaction between the manic depression and the substance misuse involves two main approaches:

■ Encourage a trial of abstinence to see how this affects the mood. There is a fair chance that, contrary to patients' expectations, abstinence actually improves mood and they gain more stability. This may be because the drug is actually worsening the mood in the longer term, even though they find it gives relief in the hours after they take it. Alternatively, the medication may prove more effective when the effect of the drugs is removed.
■ Maximise the benefits that can be obtained from the treatments for the bipolar illness, particularly the longer term preventive treatments, but commonly also treating low grade depressive symptoms. However, as with alcohol, response to treatment is often poor when the drug misuse continues.

PQ PATIENT QUESTIONS

6.27 Is it safe for me to have a baby?

The most basic question to ask about this is: 'Are you well enough to manage to take good care of yourself throughout pregnancy and yourself and your baby afterwards?' This will depend on how severe your illness is, how long you have been well for and what help and support you have from family and friends.

Pregnancy does not protect you from suffering a relapse of your bipolar illness, though the chance of this may be a bit lower. This means that most women with manic depressive illness need to take some preventive medication during pregnancy if they are going to stay well. There are some risks to the baby from you taking medicines, particularly in the first few months of pregnancy. In fact the highest risk time is the first few weeks when you may not even know that you are pregnant. That is why it is important to plan this before you get pregnant, and also when you are taking treatments that you take good contraceptive measures (*see Q. 6.14*).

6.28 What effect will the drugs I am taking have on the baby?

The great majority of babies born to women who have bipolar illness are entirely normal and only a very small proportion is affected by the type of medicine you take. However, you will need to weigh up before you get pregnant what the risks are and whether you can accept them. This is a very difficult decision to make and unfortunately many women get pregnant and then think about it, which means that they have missed the boat.

All three of the most commonly used long-term treatments (lithium, valproate and carbamazepine) can affect a baby growing inside you. Valproate and carbamazepine are particularly associated with problems in the development of the nervous system, including spina bifida, but it is likely that if you take a vitamin called folate that the risk of this occurring can be reduced. The specific risk with lithium is likely to be a heart abnormality.

It is difficult to be sure what the risk is of your baby being born with a recognisable defect. It depends on many other factors (your age, health, diet, family history) as well as the effects of any drugs. Probably the best estimate we have is that there is a 10% chance of some problems being recognised (including very minor problems) and about 1% of a severe, life-threatening problem. However, you must talk over with your doctor what the risk is in your particular case, even if in the end the doctor is not able to give you a more accurate figure.

Older antidepressant and antipsychotic drugs seem to be safer during pregnancy and some women opt to try this route of treatment.

The other side of the balance is the risk of suffering depression or mania when you are pregnant and the effect of this on your health and the medicines that you would need to take if this occurred.

6.29 Am I likely to get ill soon after I have had a baby?

You are more likely to get ill in the first few weeks after having a baby than at any other time in your life. The chance is about one in three. You should make plans to recognise this early and either take preventive treatment or have some treatment accessible to take at the first sign of illness. The chance of developing mania and psychotic symptoms (delusions and hallucinations) is particularly high.

You must tell people about this risk, including your midwife, health visitor and obstetrician, and of course your close family.

When you are pregnant you must discuss with both your general practitioner and the mental health team what you and your family should be looking out for and what medicine you should be taking. If you are not taking any medicine to prevent a recurrence of the manic depression when you are pregnant you should seriously consider starting it as soon as you have the baby, even if this does mean that you cannot breast feed.

If you can manage to get through the first 2 months without a relapse then the risk of relapse goes down to how it was before you got pregnant.

6.30 Can I still have a few beers?

The basic answer to this is yes. You do need to be cautious because alcohol can interact with medications. Many medications used to treat bipolar disorder have sedative effects and alcohol will usually exaggerate this sedation or drowsiness. A good rule of thumb is that you are likely to find that each drink is worth two compared to how it would usually affect you if you were not on the treatment. However, most longer term medications would not prevent you drinking moderate amounts of alcohol. There is an element of trial and error because individuals vary in their tolerance of alcohol and medicines. Most people manage to find whether they can tolerate reasonably a small amount of alcohol in combination with their medication. Drinking and driving is dangerous for everyone but if you are also taking medication then you are at much higher risk of having an accident and you are breaking the law if you are not capable of driving because of the combined effects of alcohol and drugs.

Alcohol and manic depression interact in other ways apart from the medication issue. About a quarter of manic depressives report serious problems with alcohol use. This may be because they are trying to 'self-medicate', i.e. they are trying to reduce their symptoms by drinking. This can be to reduce anxiety, dull depression or sedate mania. Chronic high use of alcohol runs the risk of addiction and the well-known physical and mental complications of alcoholism.

The main difficulty that people find with drinking less is that so much social life revolves around drinking alcohol and most of us like to drink as it makes social situations easier and more enjoyable. However, it is worth thinking about whether you can have some social life that does not include alcohol. Exercise and sport tend not to include alcohol (at least beforehand!) but finding good avenues to socialise that don't include alcohol can be good for your mood all round, not just because you are drinking less.

6.31 What should I tell my employer or put on a job application form?

This depends on the employer! The general advice about filling in application forms is not to write manic depression on the initial form. These forms are generally only seen by lay people who have very little understanding of the illness and so the stigma of the illness is likely to lead rapidly to rejection rather than a reasonable assessment of your abilities. On the other hand it is important to let employers know that you have been ill and what the possibility is that you might become ill again. One suggestion is to put on an initial form that you have suffered from depression and are taking medication and only go into further details when you are dealing with a doctor or nurse who is assessing your occupational fitness. Obviously with small firms there is not the same occupational health back-up and so you need to have a discussion at some point with your potential employer about your illness. In the end honesty is usually the best policy, though being cautious about how much you reveal may prove more useful in the beginning! Talking to others who have been in the same position (e.g. in groups like the Manic Depression Fellowship, see Appendix 1) is often the best way of generating ideas for dealing with this difficult area.

6.32 Why can't I think as well as I used to before I developed manic depression?

Several studies have shown that people with manic depression tend to do less well on tests of 'cognitive function', i.e. thinking skills (e.g. IQ type tests). Although on average manic depressives do less well than the general population there is a wide range (as there is in the whole population) so that many with the illness are still doing better than average.

We do not know the cause of this problem. It is possible that whatever the brain change is that causes the manic depression also causes the cognitive changes. Brain scans of people with manic depression tend on average to show more minor problems than those of other people – for example on the most sensitive magnetic scans more small areas tend to 'light up'. We do not know the meaning of this, although possibly there is a blood flow problem. However, you could not look at a scan and say 'that person has manic depression and that one does not' and there is no particular area of the brain of manic depressives on which everyone has a bright spot. Some of these differences may explain why a number of people with bipolar illness have problems with memory and concentration, even when they are not depressed or manic.

The other obvious possibility is that the medicines may affect the brain. Certainly if you get a toxic level of lithium you will be generally physically ill and you can damage the brain. This is why it is so important to monitor the levels carefully so that you never have toxic levels. On the other hand, there are some interesting studies suggesting that lithium may help to protect brain cells if they are damaged by a stroke, or even protect against Alzheimer's dementia.

The other medicines – particularly the older antipsychotics – can have effects on the brain which cause sluggish thinking which is why most patients and doctors prefer the newer antipsychotics.

What can you do about this? Probably the more episodes of illness that you have the more likely you are to suffer the 'brain' problems and so doing all you can to avoid relapse is important. Also on the general principle of 'use it or lose it', keeping your mind interested, involved and active must be worthwhile for all of us.

APPENDIX I
Useful organisations and websites

PROFESSIONAL ORGANISATIONS

American Psychiatric Association www.psych.org

The APA works to ensure humane care and effective treatment for all persons with mental disorder, including mental retardation and substance-related disorders.

British Association for Psychopharmacology

http://bap.org.uk/consensus/bipolar_disorder.html

Links to flowcharts to illustrate the evidence-based guidelines, produced in consultation with the Manic Depression Fellowship.

British Psychological Society www.bps.org.uk

For the register of chartered psychologists.

Cochrane Collaboration www.cochrane.org

The Cochrane Collaboration is an international non-profit and independent organisation, dedicated to making up-to-date, accurate information about the effects of healthcare readily available worldwide. It produces and disseminates systematic reviews of healthcare interventions and promotes the search for evidence in the form of clinical trials and other studies of interventions. The major product of the Collaboration is the Cochrane Database of Systematic Reviews which is published quarterly as part of The Cochrane Library.

Community Psychiatric Nurses Association www.cpna.org.uk

The professional association and trade union in the UK for qualified mental health nurses and students.

Mentality www.mentality.org.uk

UK charity dedicated solely to the promotion of mental health. Aims to work in partnership with organisations to form and implement mental health promotion policy at local, regional or national level.

National Electronic Library of Mental Health www.nelmh.org

Information for professionals and patients. Professional information includes a list of current research and clinical trials, with links, diagnostic criteria and evidence-based treatment summaries.

National Institute for Clinical Excellence www.nice.org.uk
NICE works on behalf of the UK National Health Service and the people who use it, making recommendations on treatments and care using the best available evidence.

National Institute of Mental Health (NIMH) www.nimh.nih.gov
US government site. Includes descriptions of anxiety, panic, and related disorders and their treatment for non-medical readers, as well as access to clinical trials and research information for the practitioner.

National Mental Health Association (NMHA) www.nmha.org
Non-profit organisation addressing all aspects of mental health and mental illness in the USA.

National Teratology Information Service
www.ncl.ac.uk/pharmsc/entis.htm
Provides information about the effects of drugs on the foetus.

Primary Care Mental Health Education (PriMHE)
The Old Stables
2a Lauren Avenue
Twickenham
Middlesex TW1 4JA
www.primhe.org
A non-profit making organisation which aims to help primary healthcare professionals deliver the best standards of mental healthcare in various ways, including educational and training initiatives, fostering and sharing of best practice, encouraging research and development, and establishing collaborative and supportive partnerships with all concerned organisations.

The Royal Australian and New Zealand College of Psychiatrists
309 La Trobe Street
Melbourne
Victoria 3000
Australia
Tel: +613 9640 0646
Fax: +613 9642 5652
Email: ranzcp@ranzcp.org
www.ranzcp.org
The Resources section provides access to medical databases, documents, external links and other resources relevant to psychiatry and mental health. A range of information on psychiatric illness and mental healthcare suitable

for allied professionals and the general public is also provided within this section.

Royal College of Psychiatrists
National Headquarters
17 Belgrave Square
London SW1X 8PG
Tel: 020 7235 2351
Fax: 020 7245 1231
Email: rcpsych@rcpsych.ac.uk
www.rcpsych.ac.uk
   The RCP website provides information on anxiety disorders, including online leaflets and fact sheets and information about sources of further help (some of which are included in this list).

United Kingdom Psychiatric Pharmacy Group www.ukppg.org.uk
   The UKPPG exists to ensure best treatment with medicines for people with mental health needs and their carers.

CLINICAL TRIALS

The Balance Trial www.psychiatry.ox.ac.uk/balance/index.html
   This large simple randomised clinical trial compared lithium and valproate semi-sodium (Depakote) combination therapy with lithium monotherapy and with valproate semi-sodium monotherapy as maintenance treatment for bipolar disorder.

Centre for Evidence-Based Mental Health www.cebmh.com
   Evidence-based mental health site, promoting and supporting the teaching and practice of evidence-based mental healthcare.

Harvard Bipolar Research Program www.manicdepressive.org
   Information on current trials, as well as resources for patients and professionals, including clinical tools such as mood charts and self-report forms to download.

PATIENT INFORMATION AND SUPPORT

Anxieties.COM www.anxieties.com
   Anxieties.COM is a self-help source for people with anxiety, panic attacks, OCD, fear of flying, and other phobias. It includes medication issues and offers books and tapes for sale. The site is by psychologist/psychiatrist R. Reid Wilson, PhD, and is based in Chapel Hill, North Carolina, USA.

Anxiety Care
Cardinal Heenan Centre
326 High Road
Ilford
Essex IG1 1QP
Tel: 020 8262 8891/2
Helpline: 020 8478 3400
Email: anxietycare@aol.com
www.anxietycare.org.uk
Anxiety Care is a charity based in East London that specialises in helping people to recover from anxiety disorder through personal recovery programmes based on self-help and supported by skilled volunteers.

Anxiety Network International www.anxietynetwork.com
The Anxiety Network, which is based in Phoenix, Arizona, USA, provides information on social anxiety disorder (social phobia), panic, and generalised anxiety disorder. The site, by Thomas A. Richards, PhD, includes a social anxiety mailing list, chat room, bookstore, question and answer pages, and related links.

Connects www.connects.org.uk
Connects is a free, linking website for mental health in general, run by the Mental Health Foundation (UK). It contains information about organisations, websites, events, and news items concerned with mental health or learning disabilities. Registration required.

Depression and Bipolar Support Alliance www.ndmda.org
Toll free (from within USA): (800) 826-3632. US patient-led organisation.

@ease
c/o Rethink
30 Tabernacle Street
London EC2A 4DD
Tel: 020 7330 9100
Fax: 020 7330 9102
email: at-ease@rethink.org
Mental health education site aimed at young adults.

Mental After Care Association (MACA)
25 Bedford Square
London WC1B 3HW
Tel: 020 7436 6194

Fax: 020 7637 1980
Email: maca-bs@maca.org.uk
www.maca.org.uk
    Provides information and services to people with mental health needs and their carers. MACA is active in the community, in hospitals and in prisons.

The Patients Association www.patients-association.com
Includes an index of links to many other patient-directed and information sites.

MENTAL HEALTH CHARITIES

Canadian Mental Health Association (CMHA) www.cmha.ca
    Canadian voluntary organisation which aims to promote the mental health of all people and to serve mental health consumers, their families and friends.

Child and Adolescent Bipolar Foundation (CABF) www.bpkids.org
    US not-for-profit organisation. Parent-led organisation offering information and support for families of sufferers of early-onset bipolar disorder.

Manic Depression Fellowship
Castle Works
21 St George's Road
London SE1 6ES
Tel: 020 7793 2600
Fax: 020 7793 2639
Email: mdf@mdf.org.uk
www.mdf.org.uk
    User-led charity. Offers a range of self-help resources and support, including a legal advice line and employment advice.

Mental Health Foundation
UK Office:
7th Floor, 83 Victoria Street
London SW1H 0HW
Tel: 020 7802 0300
Fax: 020 7802 0301
Email: mhf@mhf.org.uk
Scottish Office:
5th Floor, Merchants House
30 George Square

Glasgow G2 1EG
Tel: 0141 572 0125
Fax: 0141 572 0246
Email: scotland@mhf.org.uk
www.mentalhealth.org.uk
UK charity working in the fields of mental health and learning disabilities. Publications include newsletters, books/booklets and fact sheets on mental health issues.

Mental Health Ireland
Mensana House, 6 Adelaide Street
Dun Laoghaire, Co. Dublin
Tel: 01 284 1166
Fax: 01 284 1736
Email: information@mentalhealthireland.ie
www.mentalhealthireland.ie
Voluntary organisation aiming to actively support mental health via advocacy and a range of services and projects (most via affiliate organisations).

Mind
Granta House, 15–19 Broadway
Stratford, London E15 4BQ
Tel: 020 8519 2122
Mind Information Line: 020 8522 1728 (Greater London) or 08457 660 163 (elsewhere) (9.15 a.m. to 4.45 p.m. Monday, Wednesday and Thursday)
Email: contact@mind.org.uk
www.mind.org.uk
Mental health charity in England and Wales. Campaigns on behalf of those suffering all types of mental distress (including the Mind model for choice in primary care campaign). Also offers information (via the Mindinfoline and various publications) and support, including counselling, befriending, advocacy, employment and training schemes, and supported housing.

Organization for Bipolar Affective Disorders Society (OBAD)
1019 – 7th Ave SW
Calgary, Alberta
Canada T2P 1A8
www.obad.ca/depressioninfo.htm
Canadian charity for people with bipolar, schizoaffective disorders and unipolar depression. Local support groups and information resources, including 'Ask an expert' facility.

Praxis Mental Health
143 University Street
Belfast BT7 1HP
Tel: 028 9023 4555
Provides support services for sufferers from mental illness in Northern Ireland.

SADAssociation
PO Box 989
Steyning BN44 3HG
www.sada.org.uk
Charity offering advice and support to sufferers.

Samaritans
10 The Grove
Slough
Berks SL1 1QP
National helpline: 0345 909090
www.samaritans.org.uk
UK Helpline for anyone experiencing emotional distress. Someone to talk to in confidence 24 hours a day. Details of local branches can be found in a local telephone directory.

SANE UK
2nd Floor, Worthington House
199–205 Old Marylebone Road
London W1 5QP
Tel: 020 7375 1002 (office)
SANELINE: 0845 767 8000 (open from 12 noon until 2 a.m. every day of the year)
www.sane.org.uk
SANE is a campaigning mental health charity. Its helpline, SANELINE, gives information and support to anyone coping with mental illness.

SANE Australia
PO Box 226
South Melbourne 3205
Australia
Tel: +61 3 9682 5933
Fax: +61 3 9682 5944
Email info@sane.org
www.sane.org

National charity helping people affected by mental illness via education, information and campaigns, including StigmaWatch, which monitors the media for content stigmatising those with mental health issues.

Scottish Association for Mental Health
Cumbrae House, 15 Carlton Court
Glasgow G5 9JP
Tel: 0141 568 7000
E-mail: enquire@samh.org.uk
www.samh.org.uk
Leading mental health charity in Scotland. Provides an information service and leaflets on general mental health issues, as well as running direct services to people with mental health problems, and campaigning on policy issues.

See Me Scotland www.seemescotland.org
Award-winning Scottish campaign, run by an alliance of five Scottish mental health organisations (the Highland Users Group, National Schizophrenia Fellowship Scotland, Penumbra, the Royal College of Psychiatrists and the Scottish Association of Mental Health) to deliver Scotland's first national antistigma campaign. The 'see me' campaign urges the public to 'see the person not the label', asking them to re-think both their attitudes and their behaviour towards people with a mental health problem. As well as campaigning to end stigma and raise awareness of mental health, the website lists useful links and sources of further information.

YoungMinds
102–108 Clerkenwell Road
London EC1M 5SA
Tel: 020 7336 8445
Information line: 0800 018 2138
Fax: 020 7336 8446
www.youngminds.org.uk
Children's mental health charity. Provides confidential information service, leaflets and consultancy service.

REFERENCES, COLLECTED RESOURCES AND INTERNET PORTALS
DSM Criteria www.psychnet-uk.com/dsm_iv/dsm_iv_index.htm

World Health Report 2001: Mental health: new understanding, new hope
www.who.int/whr/2001//main/en/index.htm

BMJ collected articles http://bmj.com/cgi/collection/mood_disorders

BBC health site resources
www.bbc.co.uk/health/conditions/depression.shtml

Netdoctor http://depression.netdoctor.co.uk
Discussion boards, 'ask the expert' and news bulletins. Community developed in association with the Newcastle Affective Disorders Group at University of Newcastle.

Doctor's guide www.docguide.com
US website which gathers latest medical news and information for patients or friends/parents of patients diagnosed with depression.

Internet mental health www.mentalhealth.com
Canadian site of links to resources on various disorders – details on diagnosis, description (European, US), recent research, booklets and links to external sources of information

PsychNet-UK www.psychnet-uk.com/dsm_iv/dsm_iv_index.htm
PsychNet-UK is an independent psychology and mental health information site, run for the benefit of mental health professionals or those interested in mental health practices. It provides disorder information sheets and information on DSM-IV criteria.

Mental Help Net www.mentalhelp.net
This American 'megasite' is a comprehensive source of online mental health information, news and resources.

Shyness and Social Anxiety Service of Australia
www.socialanxiety.com.au
Providing information, education and support to consumers, carers, health practitioners and the wider community on all aspects of social anxiety disorder.

WHO Guide to Mental and Neurological Health in Primary Care
www.mentalneurologicalprimarycare.org
This guide, developed by the WHO Collaborating Centre for Research and Training for Mental Health, Institute of Psychiatry, King's College, London, is designed to assist primary care clinicians to help people with mental ill health. A brief summary of diagnosis and management is given for each condition and the management summaries include information for

the patient, advice and support, descriptions of treatment methods and indications for specialist referrals. They are supported by a linked set of resources: a mental disorder assessment guide, interactive summary cards and patient information and self-help leaflets.

JOURNALS

Acta Psychiatrica Scandinavica www.blackwellpublishing.com
American Journal of Psychiatry http://intl-ajp.psychiatryonline.org
Archives of General Psychiatry http://archpsyc.ama-assn.org
Bipolar Disorders www.blackwellpublishing.com
British Journal of Psychiatry http://bjp.rcpsych.org
Clinical Approaches in Bipolar Disorders www.bipolardisorders.net
Journal of Affective Disorders www.elsevier.com
Journal of Clinical Psychiatry www.psychiatrist.com
Journal of Clinical Psychopharmacology www.psychopharmacology.com
Journal of Psychopharmacology www.sagepub.com/journal.aspx?pid=31

APPENDIX 2
Advance directive to assist practitioners

NAME: Mrs Alexandra Owen (I prefer to be called Sandy)
ADDRESS: The Cottage, High Street, Girton, Cambridge
TELEPHONE: 01223 12345

IMPORTANT INFORMATION
PLEASE READ THE FOLLOWING STATEMENT CAREFULLY
I trust my friend Mr David Evans, who has provide me with support and who I believe should be made aware of any planned intervention to ensure my health and safety. Please also remember that Mr Evans helps me in the running of my home. Upon any future discharge from hospital I want Mr Evans to be informed of any change to my treatment plan or care needs.

HISTORY
(What I want practitioners to know about the history of my illness as distinct from what my medical records may say.)

DIAGNOSIS: Manic depression.

NOTES ABOUT MY ILLNESS:
- I have had numerous hospital admissions since 1986.
- Each time I had delusions. The nature of the delusions is my belief that I am some form of higher being like God or a Buddha. During my high spells I am convinced I am who I say I am.
- The cycle of my illness is usually that around September time I became severely depressed, this will last until around February when I usually experience a manic spell. I want you to take notice of my daughter who can see the early warning signs of me becoming high. I want you to help me at an early stage and not leave me to deteriorate (see main indicators below).
- My loss of insight (losing touch with reality) develops rapidly, i.e. within 12 to 24 hours.

WHAT I DO WHEN I BECOME HIGH
(I would not normally do the things listed below but I may give you a convincing reason when I become high as to why it is reasonable that I am doing these things now. Some of these things may be embarrassing for me to cope with when I become well again.)

MAIN INDICATORS:
- Lack of sleep. This is the most significant symptom for me. If I do not sleep for one night I am extremely active during the night. I may be going high and need your help; if I haven't slept for three nights I am high and you may not be able to catch me to give me help to prevent further deterioration.
- I will start to visit people who I do not necessary know at any time of the day or night.
- I will become overconfident, believing everyone likes me. I become talkative and outgoing.
- I become verbally and physically aggressive; this is often unpredictable.
- I wear different clothes and more make-up.
- I become vulgar in the language I use.
- I spend a lot of money on things I do not need.
- I take my clothes off anywhere.
- I become promiscuous.
- I will stop taking my ordinary medication.
- I abuse other medication and alcohol.
- I will often start to dismantle my house. Curtains will usually come down first and I will start painting.

TREATMENTS
(I have indicated below my preferences about treatments. If my condition becomes imminently life threatening I give my permission for you to use whatever treatment is deemed professionally appropriate having consulted with my daughter.)

MOOD STABILISERS:
- I am happy to take Sodium Valpour. If I have stopped taking these please put me back on them unless there is a physical reason why I should not take them.

OTHER MEDICATION:
- I realise that a major tranquilliser will usually be necessary when I am high. I have suffered severe reaction from lithium in the past. Perhaps another medication could be tried in preference. Please watch closely for any side-effects.
- I would prefer to take smaller doses of medication earlier on, rather than to have huge amounts of medication because you have left me to deteriorate.
- I do not want ECT unless as a last resort and my life is in danger. In that case I would leave the decision to my daughter and the practitioners.

- It is my strong preference to be treated at Fulbourn Hospital or an equivalent of which my daughter approves.
- It is my strong preference to be treated by Dr Hunt of Fulbourn Hospital, telephone 01223 218807 or somebody recommended by him.

FINANCIAL MATTERS
GENERAL:
- If Mr Evans has not already done so, I would want him to take responsibility for all my financial affairs while I am ill.

OTHER FINANCIAL MATTERS:
- Mr Evans is to take charge of my cheque book, benefits books.
- Where practical I should be prevented from signing any financial papers, e.g. purchase agreements.

CONTACTS
- **Consultant psychiatrist**: Dr Hunt of Fulbourn Hospital, telephone 01223 218807. I respect him and he knows my history. He is my first choice for treatment. My second choice would be someone recommended by him.
- **GP:** Dr Burroughs, Church Lane, Girton; telephone 01223 234567
- **Social worker**: My allocated social worker is Tim Clarke of Cambridge Social Services.
- **CPN**: Susan Harrison, CMHT, Cambridge; telephone 01223 345678
- **Family and friends:** The following members of my family have all seen my when I am ill. All of these members would be the best non-professionals to consult about my illness and how I am behaving differently from usual. These individuals can be contacted on the following numbers:

....
....
....

Signed   Date

Witness   Date

APPENDIX 3
Treatment with lithium

Why have I been prescribed lithium?

Lithium is used to help treat mood swings, as happens in bipolar affective disorder or manic depression. People with bipolar affective disorder have mood swings that are much more severe than the small changes in mood that everybody experiences. With bipolar affective disorder, mood may be elevated or depressed (up or down).

When the mood is extremely elevated this is called hypomania or mania. People with hypomania feel very energetic and elated but can be irritable and frustrated. They may talk very quickly, sleep very little and be full of ideas and plans. They can be described as being 'high'. Treatment is usually needed because when people are 'high' they may make poor judgements and can quickly become exhausted. Periods of depression will also occur in bipolar disorder. Symptoms include feelings of sadness, tiredness and poor sleep. Antidepressants may be required to help lessen these obviously unpleasant symptoms. Lithium helps to stabilise the mood. It reduces the highs and the lows. Lithium is also prescribed together with certain antidepressants to increase their effect when someone is suffering from severe depression.

What exactly is lithium?

Lithium is a type of salt, which can be found naturally. It has been used for over 50 years as a mood stabiliser. The trade or brand name of your lithium might be 'Priadel', 'Camcolit', 'Liskonum' or 'Li-Liquid'. Sometimes your doctor may not write the trade name of your lithium on your prescription. Always make sure you tell your pharmacist the trade name of your lithium. It's worth remembering it.

Why do I need to have some blood tests?

The first blood test is to check that it's safe for you to take lithium. Your kidneys need to be in good shape and your thyroid gland must be working properly. After about a week, you will need another blood test. This will tell the doctor if you are taking the right dose of lithium. If they are satisfied, you will only need a blood test every 3–6 months.

Is lithium safe to take?

It is usually safe to have lithium regularly as prescribed by your doctor, but it doesn't suit everyone. Let your doctor know if any of the following apply to you, as extra care may be needed:

a) if you have any other medical condition, such as myasthenia gravis or thyroid disorder, or suffer from heart or kidney trouble, or are about to undergo surgery;

b) if you are taking any other medication, especially for arthritis or heart or blood pressure problems. This includes medicine from your pharmacist, such as ibuprofen (e.g. 'Nurofen' and others), antacids containing sodium, or theophylline;

c) if you are pregnant, breast feeding, or wish to become pregnant.

What is the usual dose of lithium?

The starting dose of lithium is usually between 200 and 400 mg a day. this is usually increased to anything between 400 and 1200 mg a day.

How should I take lithium?

Look at the label on your medicine; it should have all the necessary instructions on it. Follow this advice carefully. If you have any questions, speak to your doctor or pharmacist. Most medicines are now dispensed with an information leaflet for you to read.

What should I do if I miss a dose?

Never change your dose without checking with your doctor. If you forget a dose, take it as soon as you remember, as long as it is within a few hours of the usual time.

What will happen to me when I start taking lithium?

For most people with bipolar affective disorder highs and lows occur quite rarely. Lithium should make these highs and lows less extreme or less frequent. So, it may take months or years to appreciate the beneficial effects of lithium. The best way to know whether lithium is working for you is to compare your highs and lows before and while taking it.

Unfortunately, you might get some side-effects before your mood gets any better. Most of these should go away after a few weeks. Sometimes, the amount of lithium in you body gets too high which can be dangerous. You need to be able to spot the side-effects that can mean a high level of lithium. Look at the table below. It tells you what to do if you get any side-effects. Not everyone will get the side-effects shown. There are many other possible side-effects. Ask you pharmacist, doctor or nurse if you are worried about anything else that you think might be a side-effect.

Side-effect	What is it?	What should I do if it happens to me?
COMMON		
TREMOR	Fine shaking of the hands	If it annoys you, your doctor can give you something for it. If it gets worse and spreads to the legs or jaw, stop taking you lithium and see your doctor.
STOMACH UPSET	This includes feeling and being sick and getting diarrhoea.	If it's mild, see you pharmacist. If it lasts for more than a day, stop taking your lithium and see your doctor
POLYURIA	Passing a lot of urine.	Don't drink too much alcohol. Tell your doctor about it.
POLYDIPSIA	Feeling very thirsty. Your mouth is dry and there may be a metallic taste.	Drink water or low calorie drinks in moderation. Suck boiled sweets.
LESS COMMON		
WEIGHT GAIN	Drinking more and eating more sweet things or carbohydrates.	Avoid fatty foods like chocolate, crisps and fizzy drinks. A diet full of vegetables and fibre will usually help, as will physical activities such as walking. If it becomes a problem or you are worried, ask to see a dietician.
OEDEMA	When your ankles or feet swell up.	Discuss this with your doctor when you see them next.
HYPO-THYROIDISM	Low thyroid activity – this makes you feel tired.	It's not serious. Tell your doctor the next time you see them.
RARE		
SKIN RASHES	Blotches seen anywhere.	Stop taking your lithium and see your doctor.

Signs of toxicity: your lithium level may be too high if you suffer any of the following:

- Blurred vision (things look fuzzy or you can't focus properly)
- Drowsiness or feeling sleepy or sluggish
- Confusion or slurred speech
- Increased thirst or passing more urine or water

- Dizziness and vomiting
- Unsteadiness on your feet
- Severe tremor or twitching
- Clumsiness

If these happen, stop taking it and contact your doctor now. But remember, just stopping lithium can be dangerous.

What about alcohol?

It if officially recommended that people taking lithium should not drink alcohol. This is because if both lithium and alcohol are taken at the same time, drowsiness can occur. This can lead to falls or accidents. As well as this, drinking alcohol can often make your mood unstable. Excessive drinking is especially likely to do this. Once people are used to taking medication, they can sometimes drink alcohol in small amounts without any harm. Avoid alcohol altogether for the first one or two months. After this, if you want a drink, try a glass of your normal drink and see how you feel. If this doesn't make you feel drowsy, then it is probably OK to drink small amounts. It pays to be very cautious because alcohol affects people in different ways, especially when they are taking medication.

Don't stop taking your medication because you fancy a drink at the weekend. If you do drink alcohol, drink only small amounts. Never drink any alcohol and drive while on lithium. Discuss any concerns you may have with your pharmacist, doctor or nurse.

When I feel better, can I stop taking it?

You should never stop taking lithium suddenly. People that do suddenly stop taking lithium become ill much more quickly than those who come off it slowly. Lithium is usually a long-term treatment. It is not addictive. You and your doctor should decide together when it is time for you to come off it. This should be gradually over at least 4 weeks, if not longer.

Do I need to know anything else?

Yes. The amount of salt in your diet can change the level of lithium in your body. Eat a balanced diet and don't change the amount of salt you usually have in your food. Some illnesses can change the amount of salt in our bodies. We lose salt in our sweat, and when we have a fever or 'flu. We also lose salt if we are sick or have diarrhoea. All these conditions can change the level of lithium in our bodies. Do not ignore feelings of thirst – keep up your fluid intake.

Remember, leaflets like this can only describe some of the effects of medication. You may find other books or leaflets also useful. If you have access to the Internet you may find a lot of information there as well, but be careful, as Internet-based information is not always accurate. Reproduced with permission from the United Kingdom Psychiatric Pharmacy Group, © 2001.

REFERENCES AND FURTHER READING

References

Amsterdam J, Garcia Espana F, Fawcett J et al. Efficacy and safety of fluoxetine in treating bipolar II major depression. J Clin Psychopharmacol 1998;18:435–440

Anderson I M, Nutt D J, Deakin J F. Evidence-based guidelines for treating depressive disorders with antidepressants. J Psychopharmacol 2000;14:3–20

Angst J, Gamma A. Prevalence of bipolar disorders: traditional and novel approaches. Clin Approach Bipolar Disord 2002;1:10–14

Angst J, Sellaro R. Historical perspectives and natural history of bipolar disorder. Soc Biol Psychiatry 2000;48:445–457

Bennie E H, Manzoor A K M, Scott A M, Fell G S. Serum concentrations of lithium after three proprietary preparations of lithium carbonate (Priadel, Phasal and Camcolit). Br J Clin Pharmacol 1977;4:479–483

Boniface S, Ziemann U. Plasticity in the human nervous system: investigations with transcranial magnetic stimulation. Cambridge: Cambridge University Press, 2003

Bowden C L, Calabrese J R, McElroy S L et al. A randomized, placebo-controlled 12-month trial of divalproex and lithium in treatment of outpatients with bipolar I disorder. Arch Gen Psychiatry 2000;57:481–489

Calabrese J R, Bowden C L, Sachs G S et al. A double-blind placebo-controlled study of lamotrigine monotherapy in outpatients with bipolar depression. J Clin Psychiatry 1999;60(2):79–88

Calabrese J R, Bowden C L, Sachs G S et al. A placebo-controlled 18-month trial of lamotrigine and lithium maintenance treatment in recently depressed patients with bipolar I disorder. J Clin Psychiatry 2003;64:1013–1024

Drug and Therapeutics Bulletin. Using lithium safely. DTB 1999;37(3):22–24

Freeman M P, Smith K W, Freeman S A et al. The impact of reproductive events on the course of bipolar disorder in women. J Clin Psychiatry 2002;63(4):284–287

Gershon E S, Hamovit J, Guroff J J et al. A family study of schizoaffective, bipolar I, bipolar II, unipolar and normal control probands. Arch Gen Psychiatry 1982;39:1157–1167

Goodwin G (on behalf of the BAP consensus group). Evidence based guidelines for treating bipolar disorder. J Psychopharmacol 2003;17:140–173

Gottesman I. Schizophrenia genesis: the origins of madness. New York: Freeman, 1991

Greil W, Ludwig-Mayerhofer W, Erazo N et al. Lithium versus carbamazepine in the maintenance treatment of bipolar disorders – a randomised study. J Affective Disord 1997;43:151–161

Hirschfeld R M A. The mood disorder questionnaire (MDQ). Am J Psychiatry 2000;157(11):183–185. Online: Available http://www.bipolar.com/mdq.htm

Hunt N, Bruce-Jones W, Silverstone T. Life events and relapse in bipolar affective disorder. J Affective Disord 1992;25:13–20

Isometsa E T, Henriksson M M, Aro H M, Lonnqvist J K. Suicide in bipolar disorder in Finland. Am J Psychiatry 1994;151:1020–1024

Jamison K R. Touched with fire. Manic-depressive illness and the artistic temperament. New York: Free Press Paperbacks, 1994

Lam D, Watkins E, Hayward P et al. A randomised controlled study of cognitive therapy for relapse prevention in bipolar affective disorder. Arch Gen Psychiatry 2003;60:145–152

Medicines and Healthcare Products Regulatory Agency. Interim report of the Committee on Safety of Medicines' Expert Working Group on Selective Serotonin Reuptake Inhibitors. September 2003

Monkul E S, Malhi G S, Soares J C. Mood disorders – review of structural MRI studies. Acta Neuropsychiatr 2003;15:368–380

NICE Technology Appraisal 66. Olanzapine and valproate semisodium in the treatment of acute mania associated with bipolar I disorder. Online: Available www.nice.org.uk. September 2003

Peet M. Induction of mania with selective serotonin re-uptake inhibitors and tricyclic antidepressants. Br J Psychiatry 1994;164:549–550

Prien R F, Kupfer D J, Mansky P A et al. Drug therapy in the prevention of recurrences in unipolar and bipolar affective disorders. Arch Gen Psychiatry 1984;41:1096–1104

Prien R F, Point P, Caffey E M, Klett J, Point P. Prophylactic efficacy of lithium carbonate in manic depressive illness. Arch Gen Psychiatry 1973;28:337–341

Quitkin F M, Kane J, Rifkin A, Ramos-Lorenzi J R, Nayak D V. Prophylactic lithium carbonate with and without imipramine for bipolar I patients. Arch Gen Psychiatry 1981;38:902–907

Schou M. Is there a lithium withdrawal syndrome? Br J Psychiatry 1993;163:514–518

Schou M. The effect of prophylactic lithium treatment on mortality and suicidal behaviour: a review for clinicians. J Affective Disord 1998;50:253–259

Silverstone T. Moclobemide vs. imipramine in bipolar depression: a multicentre double-blind clinical trial. Acta Psychiatr Scand 2001;104:104–109

Smoller J, Finn C. Family, twin and adoption studies of bipolar disorder. Am J Med Genet 2003;123C:48–58

Stoll A L, Severus W E, Freeman M et al. Omega 3 fatty acids in bipolar disorder: a preliminary double-blind, placebo-controlled trial. Arch Gen Psychiatry 1999;56:407–412

Suppes T, Baldessarini R J, Faedda G L, Tohen M. Risk of recurrence following discontinuation of lithium treatment in bipolar disorder. Arch Gen Psychiatry 1991;48:1082–1088

Tohen M, Chengappa K N R, Suppes T et al. Relapse prevention in bipolar I disorder: 18-month comparison of olanzapine plus mood stabiliser v. mood stabiliser alone. Br J Psychiatry 2004;184:337–345

Turner T. Anxiety: your questions answered. Edinburgh: Churchill Livingstone, 2003

Further reading

Bazire S. Psychotropic drug directory 2003. Dinton: Mark Allen Publishing, 2003
There is also a general practice version – The GP Psychotropic Handbook. Both contain a wealth of practical information on the use of drugs for psychiatric illness.

Bourne E J. The anxiety and phobia workbook. Oakland, CA: New Harbinger Publications, 2000
This is a very practical and approachable book for patients on how to manage anxiety, using cognitive and behavioural techniques.

British National Formulary, 47th edn. London: British Medical Association and the Royal Pharmaceutical Society of Great Britain, 2004
The British National Formulary is the standard reference for drug prescribing in the United Kingdom and has detailed advice on prescribing, including information on drug interactions and pregnancy.

Clare A, Milligan S. Depression and how to survive it. New York: Random House, 1993
An account from the inside (by Spike Milligan) and the outside by Professor Clare which is both readable and informative.

Cookson J, Taylor D, Katona C. Use of drugs in psychiatry. London: Royal College of Psychiatrists, 2002
The latest edition of a classic guide to prescribing in psychiatry. It manages to cover a broad spectrum of conditions but also gives detailed advice on all the medicines you are likely to use.

Goodwin F K, Jamison K R. Manic depressive illness. New York: Oxford University Press, 1990
This is the standard detailed textbook on manic depression. Although it is now more than 10 years old it still provides a sound academic basis for understanding and treating bipolar disorder.

Greenberger D, Padesky C. Mind over mood. London: Guilford Press, 1995
A self-help book based on a cognitive therapy approach for patients in improving depression.

Jamison K R. An unquiet mind. A memoir of moods and madness. London, Picador, 1996
A biographical view of manic depression from a psychologist (and author of the major textbook). Although essentially the story of her life, her expertise gives an extra dimension to the book.

Sachs G S. Bipolar mood disorder: practical strategies for acute and maintenance phase treatment. J Clin Psychopharmacol 1996;16(2 Suppl 1): 32S–47S
There is a downloadable monthly mood chart available at http://psycheducation.org/ PCP/handouts/Mood_Chart.doc based on this research.

LIST OF PATIENT QUESTIONS

INDEX

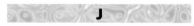
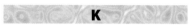
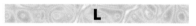